HEAL YOUR RELATIONSHIP WITH FOOD

JULIET ROSEWALL,

AMY CHISHOLM

AND MAUREEN MOERBECK

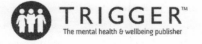

TRIGGER™
The mental health & wellbeing publisher

First published in Great Britain 2020 by Trigger

Trigger is a trading style of Shaw Callaghan Ltd & Shaw Callaghan 23 USA, INC.

The Foundation Centre

Navigation House, 48 Millgate, Newark

Nottinghamshire NG24 4TS UK

www.triggerpublishing.com

British Library Cataloguing in Publication Data

A CIP catalogue record for this book is available upon request from the British Library

ISBN: 9781789561272

This book is also available in e-Book format:

ePUB: 9781789561289

Cover design by Georgie Hewitt

Typeset by Lapiz Digital Services

Printed and bound in Great Britain by CPI Group (UK) Ltd, Croydon CRO 4YY

Paper from responsible sources

CONTENTS

MEET THE AUTHORS

DR JULIET ROSEWALL

Juliet Rosewall is a Health and Care Professions Council (HCPC) registered Clinical Psychologist currently working in an NHS Child and Adolescent Eating Disorders service in London. She has experience in the assessment and treatment of eating-related problems in young people and adults, and has worked in the field of mental health, in both research and clinical roles, for the last 20 years.

Juliet trained at the University of Canterbury, in New Zealand. Following the completion of her PhD and clinical psychology training in 2009, Juliet worked at an eating disorders service and child and adolescent mental health service in New Zealand. She moved to the UK in 2010 and, since this time, has worked with adults with eating disorders and, more recently, children and adolescents in both general mental health and eating disorder settings. As well as her clinical work, Juliet is research active, and trains and regularly supervises others in their clinical practice.

Juliet strongly believes in providing specialised evidence-based psychological treatments through utilising a warm and compassionate approach. She is passionate about working collaboratively with those she treats, in order to bring about meaningful change to their eating behaviours and body image. She believes that there is hope for those who are struggling with an eating problem and it is fully possible to move towards a valued life that is not ruled by food, eating or appearance.

AMY CHISHOLM

Amy Chisholm is a Clinical Psychologist registered with the Health and Care Professions Council in the UK. Amy has worked in adult mental health for eighteen years, and the field of eating disorders for seventeen years. Amy has worked since 2012 in specialist eating disorders services for adults in the UK in both the National Health Service (NHS) and a private capacity. Amy worked for a number of years in a large specialist eating disorders service in London as a Clinical Psychologist, offering individual therapy and supervising junior colleagues. Amy also specialises in treatment of trauma-related problems, and works in specialist NHS trauma services for adults.

Amy is originally from New Zealand and trained at the University of Canterbury. In 2008 she completed her Master of Arts in Psychology and in 2009 her Postgraduate Diploma in Clinical Psychology. Since this time Amy has also completed a Postgraduate Diploma in Cognitive Behavioural Therapy through the University of Otago in New Zealand. She has also completed her two-year training in Cognitive Analytic Therapy and is registered with the Association for Cognitive Analytic Therapy in the UK.

Amy enjoys working with people experiencing eating problems, having repeatedly seen the power of noticing and breaking destructive cycles of eating that people naturally fall into. Amy whole-heartedly believes that change is possible and loves to help people find new ways of seeing things, new ways of doing things, and new ways of relating to themselves that will help them be free to live the life they truly want to live.

MAUREEN MOERBECK

Originally from Australia, Maureen graduated with an honours degree in Nutrition & Dietetics in 2003 and moved to the UK in 2006. She is a registered dietitian with the Health and Care Professions Council (HCPC) and is a member of the British Dietetic Association (BDA), the London Eating Disorders

Dietitians Group, The Centre for Mindful Eating, and the Health At Every Size (HAES) community.

She works for an NHS Eating Disorders Service in London and has worked with adult and adolescents in outpatient, day patient and inpatient settings. In addition, Maureen has her own private practice called Mindful Nutrition Practice, where she supports clients with eating disorders and disordered eating. She also works for BEAT (the UK's national eating disorders charity) as a Clinical Associate Trainer where she delivers training to schools.

Whilst working for the NHS, she has completed a Diploma in Sports Nutrition with the International Olympic Committee, a Graduate Certificate in Public Health, has trained in mindful eating and has recently become a qualified meditation teacher.

Maureen studied Nutrition & Dietetics with the hope of being able to support clients with eating disorders in their work towards recovery. After eight years of working as a dietitian in a variety of clinical settings, she moved towards specialising in eating in 2011 and has been practising in this setting since then.

Maureen is passionate about helping people throughout their journey of recovery. This includes helping clients return to normal eating, debunking nutrition and diet culture myths, rediscovering their own internal cues and improving their relationship with food and their body using a Non-Diet and HAES approach.

INTRODUCTION

Food. It is a part of all of our lives and a basic need for survival. It is necessary for our growth and strength. It is also a part of how we enjoy life and connect with others. Despite this, many people struggle with their relationship with food and can develop all-consuming problems with this vital aspect of life.

Eating problems can take many different forms. You may constantly want to diet, or find yourself focused on "clean" eating or weight loss, despite this focus making you unhappy and preoccupied. Or you may have issues with eating past comfortable fullness, feeling out of control when you eat, or finding that you eat in response to emotions. Other people use extreme behaviours to manage feelings of fear or guilt about eating, such as vomiting, driven exercise, misusing laxatives or taking diet pills. Often these eating problems start in an effort to feel better about some aspect of life – but few people feel happy about being so preoccupied with eating! Not to mention the physical and psychological consequences that can be a result.

If you have picked up this book, we think that you (or someone you care about) may be finding these various forms of eating problems distressing, exhausting, frustrating – and getting in the way of living the life you want to live.

Eating problems often develop gradually. They may start with small changes here and there in your attitudes and behaviours towards food. Before you know it, these thoughts and eating behaviours can start to cause problems in your life.

Some of the common signs that you might be developing problems with eating include:

- Worrying about food and eating-related situations
- Guilt or fear about eating
- Episodes of being unable to stop eating ("binge eating")
- Rapid weight changes
- Avoiding situations involving food, such as social outings or birthdays
- Having black-and-white rules about eating that mustn't be broken
- Becoming consumed with thoughts about food
- Noticing or talking about body weight and shape a lot
- Weighing yourself repeatedly
- Obsessively counting calories or trying to restrict your calories to a certain number
- Feeling as though you need to earn the right to eat
- Attempting to "compensate" for eating by vomiting, using diet pills, laxatives, or exercising in a driven way
- Avoiding entire food groups
- Finding that your mood, life satisfaction and self-worth depend on eating and your weight

As with overcoming any problem behaviour, we believe that early awareness and acknowledgement of the problem is important. Once you have made this first step, we would like to help you make the changes necessary to tackle your eating problems and improve your general wellbeing. We hope that this book will help you to do this.

MEET CLARE, SUKI AND CHRIS

Throughout this book we refer to three "clients": Clare, Suki and Chris. These are not specific, real-life clients, but characters based on our collective clinical experience, and they each represent common experiences we see in relation to eating problems. Have a read and take note of any aspects of their stories that you identify with.

Clare is a 20-year-old university student who constantly diets and follows various eating trends in order to lose weight. She avoids sugar and high-fat foods, tries to eat 1,500 calories a day and prefers to eat "clean". Being thin is extremely important to her and always has been. She associates thinness with being successful and achieving. She regularly weighs herself in an effort to control her weight. Clare is a self-confessed "perfectionist" and never feels she does a good enough job. She can recall times in her early childhood when she was teased about her weight and feels this has had a big impact on her life. Clare's friends think she is a bit obsessed with exercise, but Clare is not sure.

Suki is 39 and is trying to lose weight through excessive dieting. At times, she will skip meals and under-eat in the day in an attempt to lose weight. Suki will then sometimes binge eat at night on foods in the cupboard, or the leftovers of her children's dinner. She feels guilty that she cannot stick to her weight-loss plan and feels as if she "blows it" by bingeing. She has tried periods of exercising in a driven way to manage her weight, but ends up feeling exhausted. She has even vomited on two occasions in the past year as she felt so riddled with guilt after eating. She continues the cycle the next day, promising herself that she will be "better" and follow her diet again. She acknowledges that this cycle of dieting, and feeling like she is failing at it, is seriously getting her down.

Chris is a 27-year-old teacher who is struggling with eating in an out-of-control way. He eats in response to his emotions, especially after a stressful day at work or if there is tension with his partner. Eating helps Chris reduce his feelings of stress and sadness, but afterwards he feels even worse, as if he has failed. Chris feels ashamed about his eating and is very secretive about it. Chris realises his eating has become out of control, but he feels stuck – unsure about how to move forward.

You may relate to aspects of one or two of these people, though it's likely that your eating problems may be slightly different. As we shall see, eating problems can come in various forms, with similarities and differences, but regardless of the specific eating behaviours, allowing food and eating to control your life, and being consumed by shape and weight, rarely leads to contentment or fulfilment.

"Allowing food and eating to control your life, and being consumed by shape and weight, rarely leads to contentment or fulfilment."

HOW THIS BOOK CAN HELP

This is a book to help adults overcome eating problems. We will provide information on specific eating problems, how they start, and the factors that contribute to them being maintained. We will provide up-to-date information on nutrition and dieting. Following this, we will introduce well-established and time-tested techniques that we have learned and used in our work. We discuss the ideas we have found most helpful for the many people we have helped with eating problems. These include skills and techniques to help you think differently about food, eating, emotions and your body.

If you are a clinician, there are a number of excellent textbooks we recommend, which have inspired many of the ideas in this book (see Useful Resources section at the end). We hope to make the ideas that we have learned and practised over the years, accessible for readers at home.

WHEN TO GET PROFESSIONAL HELP

This book is not a diagnostic manual and is not a substitute for tailored, face-to-face therapy with a specialist or registered health professional.

Left untreated, eating problems can increase in severity and frequency and may deteriorate into a full-blown eating disorder, such as Anorexia Nervosa, Bulimia Nervosa or Binge Eating Disorder.

Anorexia Nervosa is characterised by the restriction of food intake leading to a low weight (defined as less than minimally normal, or what one would expect for age, sex, developmental trajectory and physical health). It involves intense fear of weight gain, or behaviour that prevents weight gain. It also involves disturbance in body image or lack of awareness of the seriousness of the problem. Self-worth is often disproportionately based on shape and weight.

Bulimia Nervosa involves episodes of eating a large amount of food in a short period of time, that others would agree is large, and feeling out of control during this time. People describe this "out of control" feeling as an inability to stop once they start eating. This is also known as binge eating. Someone with Bulimia Nervosa would also try to "compensate" for the food they have eaten (for example by vomiting, misusing laxatives or excessively exercising). Like Anorexia, self-worth is based disproportionately on shape and weight. To receive a formal diagnosis, these episodes need to occur once a week for at least three months.

Finally, **Binge Eating Disorder** is characterised by the presence of regular binge eating (as seen with Bulimia), but without compensatory behaviours. Binge eating is accompanied by significant distress, and three of the following: eating more rapidly than normal; eating until uncomfortably full; eating large amounts of food when not physically hungry; eating alone because of feeling embarrassed by the amount of food; and feeling disgusted, depressed or very guilty afterwards. Like Bulimia, these episodes occur at least once a week for at least three months to warrant diagnosis.

If you identify with any of the above descriptions, please seek help from a doctor or a psychologist for an assessment, diagnosis, and to discuss treatment options. In particular, if you are significantly underweight and have noticed physical impacts (such as feeling faint or dizzy, or not menstruating), then *act now*. We recommend that you see your doctor for an assessment of your physical health and to seek a referral from your GP or doctor to an appropriate specialist eating disorders service for face-to-face treatment.

Eating disorders are best treated as soon as possible, so we urge you to seek help quickly from an appropriately trained professional.

EATING PROBLEMS IN YOUNG PEOPLE

Please note, the approach used with young people with eating problems is different and should generally involve working with the family. If you are under eighteen years of age, or if you are an adult worried about a young person, please contact your GP or doctor for a referral to an appropriate local child and adolescent eating disorders or mental health service (CAMHS in the UK) for guidance, or look for a therapist with experience in family-based approaches to treating adolescent eating problems.

CARING FOR A LOVED ONE WITH AN EATING PROBLEM

If you have picked up this book because someone you love has an eating problem, we hope you will find it a useful guide to understand what they might be going through and what strategies may help them. If you are looking for a carer-specific guide, please see our recommended reading at the back of this book.

PART I

THE GROUNDWORK

CHAPTER 1

UNDERSTANDING YOUR EATING PROBLEMS

The first step to healing your relationship with food is to take some time to fully understand your eating problems. This includes exploring your specific eating behaviours, what function they play in your life now, and what keeps them going.

Eating problems often begin gradually. Before long you might find yourself stuck in a pattern of behaviour, not quite understanding how this all came about. Everyone who struggles with their eating is different and will have their own unique reasons for having a problematic relationship with food. You might have even tried to make changes but then feel overwhelmed with the task ahead, or unsure how to change. There are lots of very good reasons why eating problems start, and very understandable reasons that they continue.

In this section we will shine a light on these reasons, in the hope that you no longer feel you are fumbling in the dark

"Is it your body that needs to change, or your mindset?"

for a way forward. We will focus on the factors that are keeping your eating problems going in the here and now, as this is going to be the most important place to make changes. Of course, it is understandable to be curious about the historical reasons for your eating problems, and sometimes this knowledge can be helpful (we will touch on this later). However, as hard as it can sometimes be to accept, we cannot change the past. But we *can* change our present and future, so this is where we will focus.

To begin, let's look at three groups of eating problems – dieting, binge eating and compensatory behaviours – and some of the most common reasons for them.

DIETING

"Dieting" describes the restriction of calories and/or specific foods/food groups to change or maintain body shape or weight. Changing the way we eat to improve nutritional balance can be beneficial for health. However, a large amount of research demonstrates that dieting (restricting your eating) is detrimental to one's emotional and physical wellbeing. Moreover, the weight loss that occurs as a result of dieting is generally fleeting, with weight regain to, or above, the original level being the norm.[1] In short, diets don't work. So why do some people continue to diet?

"In short, diets don't work."

PLACING DISPROPORTIONATE IMPORTANCE ON YOUR SHAPE AND WEIGHT

People often diet because body shape and weight are extremely important to them. Given our society's current focus on body shape, striving for thinness, muscularity and muscle tone has become a pursuit for many. If your body's shape and weight is a significant marker of achievement or happiness for you, dieting may have been a way to feel happy or proud. However, the constant pressure of dieting often leads to increased body preoccupation, feeling hungry and feeling unhappy.

In this situation, ask yourself: is it your body that needs to change, or your mindset?

---

[1] Mann, T., Tomiyama, A. J., Westling, E., Lew, A.-M., Samuels, B., & Chatman, J. (2007). Medicare's search for effective obesity treatments: Diets are not the answer. *American Psychologist, 62*(3), 220–233. doi.org/10.1037/0003–066X.62.3.220

FEAR OF FATNESS

Sadly, in many Western societies there is a preoccupation with thinness. Many people grow up with message that "thin = good" and "fat = bad". From a young age, we learn from our families, the media and our peers that it is inherently bad to gain weight. While it is true that there are health consequences to obesity, our society has a strong focus on the consequences of obesity and less of a focus on the consequences of under-eating and being under-weight. It is also the case that a bombardment of negative information and pressure to avoid obesity often paralyses people rather than helping to prompt a balanced eating pattern.

Just because someone is in a larger body doesn't automatically mean they are unhealthy, or that their health is affected by their weight. There are so many factors *other* than weight that determine whether someone is in good health or not. In fact, sometimes it is the actual *fear* of fatness that can fuel unhealthy cycles of dieting behaviour and subsequent poor health.

MISUNDERSTANDING NORMAL BODY CHANGES

There is a myth in our society that we can completely control our weight. For some, this leads to excessive monitoring of changes in weight or body shape, for example by weighing yourself on a daily basis or checking yourself in the mirror throughout the day. People might then react to normal fluctuations in weight or body shape, misinterpreting them as permanent. In fact, it is normal for our weight and body shape to fluctuate on a daily basis (more on this in Chapter 17) and misinterpreting these normal fluctuations can drive dieting behaviour.

NEEDING CONTROL

Another reason many people diet is to gain a feeling or perception of control. Many people with eating problems talk about how dieting helps when other aspects of their lives feel uncontrollable. Temporary control over one's eating can give some short-term relief from feelings or situations that are overwhelming. This might be conflict at home or work, financial trouble, academic pressures or relationship problems.

While trying to control your eating, you may have found that your eating problem has begun to control you. For example, say you have been invited out for

"Ask yourself: who is really in control?" dinner with your friends to a local pizza restaurant, but you are avoiding carbohydrates, and therefore pizza is a forbidden food for you. Despite friendships and celebrating being important to you, you decide not to go. Your effort to avoid carbohydrates in order to feel better about yourself is actually limiting your ability to be with your friends and have an enjoyable evening. If you relate to this, ask yourself: who is really in control?

PRESSURE FROM OTHERS

Perhaps you diet because others have made comments about your appearance and you are feeling pressure to lose weight. Research tells us that those who experience pressure to diet or to lose weight from friends, family and the media are more likely to feel dissatisfied with their shape and weight.[2] This, in turn, can lead to eating problems. Have a think: are there people in your life that make you feel pressured in this way? If so, can you have a conversation with them about how their comments are affecting you? If this doesn't work, think about your personal boundaries and whether distancing yourself from these people or sources, even temporarily, might be the best way forward.

---

[2]   Stice, E. (2002). Risk and maintenance factors for eating pathology: A meta-analytic review. *Psychological Bulletin*, 128, 825–848.

BINGE EATING

As mentioned, binge eating (or bingeing) describes the behaviour of eating in an out of control way, often experienced as being unable to stop once you start. Whilst some people binge on an amount of food that is objectively large, others might binge on an amount of food that *feels* excessive but is a normal-sized amount of food. The sense of loss of control is a key feature of bingeing. Binge eating can be really upsetting and have a negative impact on one's life, yet can be a very difficult habit to break. So why do some people continue to binge?

UNDER-EATING

More often than not, people binge eat because they haven't eaten enough in the day. Research shows that very often binges are a result of not eating sufficient calories or restricting food intake in the day. People may under-eat in an effort to lose weight. Or maybe they do so accidentally because they're not paying enough attention to the amount and types of food they're eating. For example, after a busy day at work, having not eaten enough, you are ravenous when you get home. There is a simple biology behind this: your blood sugar levels have dropped significantly and your body is craving the energy it needs.

BREAKING THE "RULES"

When someone is dieting, they often have strict rules about what and how much they "should" eat. For example, "I must not eat after 8pm", "I must only eat raw, unrefined foods" or "I must avoid cake". Now, rules are different to guidelines (more on that later), but, as the saying goes, rules are made to be broken. Human beings are inherently rebellious. There is something in our mind that wants to break a rule that is imposed on us. This is the same with our eating. After a period of dieting or avoiding certain foods, you might experience a "Sod it" or "I give up" moment, whereby you binge eat these "forbidden" foods.

Often eating your forbidden foods is followed by the experience of guilt (for breaking a rule) or fear of the consequences (e.g. fear of weight gain). This might lead to a renewed motivation to continue your dieting and avoidance of these foods, thereby maintaining the problem. In these instances, you might have thought, "I just need to try harder next time" or "I have no self-control". In fact, what you are trying to fight is your biology and basic human needs, so "self-control" isn't the answer. It is important, therefore, to see dieting as the *problem*, not the solution.

"It is important to see dieting as the *problem*, not the solution."

EMOTIONAL EATING

Many people change their eating in response to their emotions. It is common to eat when we are happy, to celebrate. Food is rewarding in that way. It is also common to eat when we are sad, to commiserate. While this is a normal part of life, it becomes an issue if your main or only way of coping with your emotions is to eat past comfortable fullness or under-eat, as you may find that your eating becomes out of control during times of intense emotion.

Sometimes people also binge eat as a way to completely block unwanted emotions. Bingeing might serve to distract you from your feelings, or even serve to temporarily shut them down altogether, although they usually come back, even stronger unfortunately (more on this in Chapter 16).

You might also find you are binge eating to experience feelings of pleasure in a day that is otherwise full of stress, worry or other negative feelings. Sometimes, when life feels difficult, a chance to eat something enjoyable can seem like your only opportunity for pleasure in a day. This is completely understandable – we all need to have some pleasure in our lives! – but it becomes a problem when eating is your *main* or *only* source of pleasure. If this is the case, it is important to look at what else you need in your life so that pleasure from eating remains enjoyable, but your emotional wellbeing is not dependent on it.

DISINHIBITION
Sometimes in life we find ourselves on autopilot. At these times you will have less ability to reflect on your behaviour and make proactive choices. These occasions might be due to tiredness, stress or the effects of using alcohol or drugs. It could also be because you are preoccupied with something, or you are simply zoned out watching your favourite box set. We will talk about mindful eating later, but for now, try to recognize that acting on autopilot will lead to a reduced ability to tune in to your internal cues, notice what you really need or want, and make thoughtful choices.

COMPENSATORY BEHAVIOURS
"Compensatory behaviours" are strategies people use after eating, in an effort to prevent weight gain, or counteract fullness or emotional responses to eating. After eating past fullness, you might experience a variety of thoughts and feelings, such as "I shouldn't have done that", "I'm out of control" or "I'm going to put on so much weight". You might also feel emotions like guilt, fear and regret; or physical sensations such as fullness, bloating, nausea and tightness in your clothes.

You might find yourself looking for ways to counteract these unpleasant experiences by trying to compensate for the eating behaviour, such as exercising in a driven way, fasting, vomiting, or using laxatives or diet pills. These behaviours usually bring short-term relief from feeling guilty or sick, which is why you might have found it hard to change these behaviours on your own.

Unfortunately, as well as the relief being short-lived, there are longer-term negative effects. Compensatory behaviours rarely have the effects on weight you might have hoped and tend to

"Compensatory behaviours rarely have the effects on weight you might have hoped and tend to leave you feeling unhappy or exhausted."

leave you feeling unhappy or exhausted. Ultimately, the behaviours can become entrenched and you might use them as a kind of permission to binge in the first place, i.e. "It's okay to binge eat now because I will go for a really long run/vomit/fast/take a laxative later". This pattern of problematic eating and attempting to compensate can become habitual, and in this way compensatory behaviours only become an additional problem for you to deal with, rather than the solution you had hoped for.

Now we have identified some of the reasons people find themselves with these behaviours, we are going to dig deep into what keeps them going, how ready you are to change these behaviours, and how you can change them. Before we do so, let's take a look at what our body needs to function and debunk some myths that might be driving your eating problem.

CHAPTER 2

YOUR BODY'S NUTRITIONAL NEEDS

Sometimes we get so lost in misconceptions about food and eating that we lose track of the basic fact that food is *critical for survival*. You need a range of food to give your body the energy it requires to function optimally. Food is not "nice to have" or a treat to be enjoyed. It is vital.

With such a vast array of nutritional information out there, it is not surprising many of us feel that the only way to be healthy is to focus on eating perfectly. However, nutrition is only half of the picture when it comes to eating. Our relationship with food also matters. Even if we were eating the "perfect" amounts of every nutrient (if there were such a thing), but it would result in us overthinking everything we ate,

> "Food is not 'nice to have' or a treat to be enjoyed. It is *vital*."

banning foods we think don't fit this perfect picture, never eating food for pleasure, or avoiding eating out with others for fear of how the food is prepared. This does not equal a good relationship with food, and therefore does not equal health.

NUTRITION MYTHS AND REALITIES

If you pay attention to the media, you will see that there is an ever-changing list of nutrients or foods that are demonised or glorified on a day-to-day basis. This can leave us feeling confused and makes it difficult to know what is okay to eat. Although our body requires a wide range of vitamins and minerals for health, we can get these quite easily when we eat a good variety of foods and do not exclude any food groups from our diet.

The motto "everything in moderation" rings true here. Despite it not having the marketing appeal of most of the diets out there, it is the way to get to a *balanced*, *intuitive* and *healthy* relationship with food.

WHAT DOES OUR BODY NEED?

The information we present here is not another diet to help you lose weight. We want to help guide you towards a healthy and sustainable relationship with food. If you find yourself being sceptical, anxious or even rolling your eyes, we ask that you suspend your search for the next perfect diet for now, and give yourself an opportunity to think differently about food.

When we refer to nutrients in food, we talk about macronutrients and micronutrients.

Macronutrients are those that provide us with energy, i.e. carbohydrates, protein and fats.

Micronutrients are those that do not provide energy but provide other nutrients, i.e. vitamins, like A, B (B_1, B_2, B_3 etc.), C, D, E and K, and minerals such as calcium, iron, zinc and potassium.

A balanced diet is important for your body to get the macronutrients and micronutrients it needs. Trying to include a balance of macronutrients – carbohydrate, protein, fat – as well as fruit/vegetables enables you to nourish your body. When eaten together, they also help you feel more satisfied, as each of these groups has a different function. Eating a balanced diet is also important to prevent you from depriving yourself of something you need (be it for nutrition or enjoyment!). Deprivation is a factor that will keep an eating problem going (more on that later).

In essence, balanced eating means eating regularly, eating a full variety of foods, and not excluding or banning foods. Here is a rough idea of what your plate should contain for each meal (with examples):

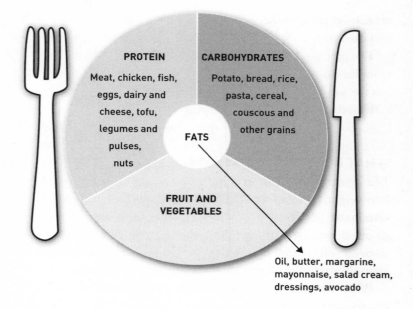

PROTEIN

Meat, chicken, fish, eggs, dairy and cheese, tofu, legumes and pulses, nuts

CARBOHYDRATES

Potato, bread, rice, pasta, cereal, couscous and other grains

FATS

FRUIT AND VEGETABLES

Oil, butter, margarine, mayonnaise, salad cream, dressings, avocado

Remember that the above diagram is a guide and does not need to be followed perfectly. Use it instead to help you notice if you are avoiding eating in this balanced way. Ask yourself:

- Am I generally including all four components in my meals? Or am I consistently avoiding one or two?
- Am I giving myself similar quantities of carbohydrate, protein and vegetables? Or am I giving myself more of one and less of another?
- Am I generally feeding myself enough of each component so that my meals satisfy me? Or am I consciously giving myself small portions, leaving me unsatisfied, wanting more, or feeling out of control later?

If you answered "no" to any of these questions, spend some time reflecting on this. By exploring why you are making these decisions, you can identify what the barriers to balanced eating are for you.

MACRONUTRIENTS

Now let's have a closer look at each of the macronutrients in detail.

CARBOHYDRATE

Carbohydrates get a bad (w)rap (no pun intended!) these days. For some reason, they have been all but demonised. Through misleading claims that continue to be repeated and embellished, carbohydrates are often believed to be the sole culprit for all that is wrong with our health. However, this could not be further from the truth.

> **"Carbohydrates are often believed to be the sole culprit for all that is wrong with our health. However, this could not be further from the truth."**

Reasons we need carbohydrate:

- To give us energy
- To keep our mood stable
- To aid clarity of thought
- To help with regular bowel movements
- To ensure our metabolism is working at its optimal level

Here are two common statements you may hear with regard to carbohydrates:

1. "Carbohydrates are bad because they make you gain weight"
2. "Carbohydrates are just sugar, and sugar is unhealthy"

Both are myths. Let us explain why…

/

Myth 1: "Carbohydrates are bad because they make you gain weight"

Well, let's look at this a bit closer. To do this, it is worth understanding how carbohydrate is broken down in the body. Carbohydrate is made up of molecules of sugar (don't freak out yet!). These can be monosaccharides (one sugar), disaccharides (two sugars), oligosaccharides (a few sugars), or polysaccharides (many sugars). Monosaccharides and disaccharides are often termed "simple" sugars, whereas oligosaccharides and polysaccharides are often called "starches" or "complex" carbohydrates. When we eat carbohydrate, our body breaks down the carbohydrate into its most basic unit – the monosaccharide.

All carbohydrates, no matter whether it's sugar, fruit, pasta or quinoa, are broken down and absorbed into the bloodstream in the same way. The only difference between them is how quickly this is done, i.e. how much breaking down needs to happen. Simply put, the more complex the carbohydrate is, the longer it will take for your body to digest and absorb.

When glucose (sugar) is absorbed into the bloodstream, it triggers a hormone called insulin to be released. Insulin acts like a key. It essentially opens up the cells within our body (mainly muscle and liver cells) so that the glucose is able to enter. This is how energy is made.

Insulin also helps us store up glucose as "glycogen". These glycogen stores are vital, as they allow us to draw on a reserve of energy any time we need it (without having to eat constantly). So, when someone has not been eating enough carbohydrate, there will be little to no glycogen stores. The important point here is that when glycogen is stored, water is stored alongside it. The more glycogen is stored, the more water there will be. This is why people might notice their weight drop after they eat a low carbohydrate diet. It's not because they've actually lost weight (i.e. fat), but because they have depleted their vital glycogen stores and the associated water.

Myth 2: "Carbohydrates are just sugar, and sugar is unhealthy"

As we've just established, *we need carbohydrates for energy.* We now know that sugar (glucose) is just the broken-down version of carbohydrate, and glucose is vital in the production of energy. In fact, it is the only energy source from our food that our brain uses. Did you know that your brain needs 120g carbohydrate to function? That equates to 6–8 slices of bread – and that's just for your brain! We're not even counting the energy the rest of your body needs. Without carbohydrate, therefore, we feel tired and find it difficult to concentrate – both common side effects of low-carbohydrate diets.

We also need carbohydrates to protect our muscles and metabolism. Remember, carbohydrates are our preferred source of energy. If we are not getting enough, our body needs to get them from somewhere, and that somewhere will be from our body's own stores and tissues.

"By eating carbohydrate, we keep our metabolism from slowing down."

To ensure that our body's protein (muscle and organs) is not broken down to use as an energy source, we need to be eating carbohydrate to provide that energy, thereby protecting our muscle. Muscle is a big determinant of our metabolism. By eating carbohydrate, therefore, we keep our metabolism from slowing down.

We need carbohydrates to regulate our mood. Ever wonder why cake, chocolate or just carbohydrates in general make us happy? It's not just that they're delicious; there is also a chemical explanation. As you now know, when we eat carbohydrates, insulin is released. Insulin not only allows glucose to enter our cells, it also helps amino acids to be absorbed by the muscles to help synthesise protein. Insulin is vital to give the full range of amino acids a chance to be used. This includes an amino acid called tryptophan, which has to travel to the brain to be converted into serotonin while the other amino acids are busy being absorbed by the muscles. Healthy levels of serotonin are important for mood, managing cravings, increasing pain tolerance, and sleep regulation. Low levels of serotonin can cause low mood, food cravings, insomnia and increased pain sensitivity. If we didn't eat carbohydrate, insulin wouldn't be released, and therefore there would be no serotonin produced. So, is it really that surprising that we might feel low and have cravings when we cut out carbs, or that when we feel low, we often crave carbs?

Where do we get carbohydrates from?

- Bread
- Potatoes
- Pasta
- Rice
- Grains like couscous, quinoa, polenta and bulgur wheat
- Cereals
- Legumes and pulses
- Sugar

PROTEIN

While carbohydrate is often portrayed as the villain in the food story, protein is often portrayed as the hero. So much so that we are told that we need to eat more of it, often to the detriment of other nutrients. Yes, protein is important, but it is no more important than carbohydrate or fat.

Protein is made up of amino acids, and our body requires twenty different ones for health. Some of these are made by our body, but others we need to get from food. So, it is important that we eat a varied diet to get all of our protein needs. This can be quite easy to do if we eat a broad range of protein foods (including meat), while getting all of the necessary amino acids from a plant-based diet can be more challenging. When we are in a starved state, the number of amino acids that our body makes decreases, so the number we need to get from food increases. This means that among those who are dieting, it is even more important to increase the variety of protein consumed, especially for those on a plant-based diet.

Reasons we need protein:

- To help with growth and repair of our body's muscle, tendons, skin, hair and nails
- To ensure we have a healthy immune system
- To aid digestion as the digestive enzymes contain amino acids which come from protein
- To provide the building blocks of hormones, which are needed to regulate our body's processes i.e. telling each part of your body what work to do, when to do it, and for how long
- To provide other important minerals such as iron, zinc and calcium (more on calcium and iron later on)

Where do we get protein from?

- Red meat such as beef, lamb and pork
- Chicken
- Fish and seafood
- Eggs
- Dairy
- Legumes and pulses
- Soya products including tofu
- Nuts and seeds
- Meat substitutes such as Quorn

Substituting carbohydrates for protein (or fat)?

Some diets recommend increasing protein or fat at the expense of carbohydrate. The use of protein shakes is often seen and promoted in gyms because of the belief that if protein helps build muscle, then have more protein... right?

The reality is that more protein does not equal more muscle. Our body can only use a finite amount of protein for building muscle; the excess will either be stored as fat or result in problems such as compromised physical performance, brain fog, digestive issues and bad breath. This kind of diet might also make you feel fuller for longer but may not leave you satisfied and instead trigger sugar cravings because your body is trying to receive that preferred source of energy. If we are eating a balanced and varied diet with regular protein at meals, this is often enough. There is no need for protein supplements or to add extra protein.

FATS

Fats have come back full circle recently. Ten or twenty years ago, fats were demonised and blamed for weight gain and ill health. There was a push to choose low-fat products and exclude fats as much as possible. Although this is still often followed, fat seems to have redeemed itself somewhat, and although not seen as the hero, it is perhaps now thought of as the hero's trusty sidekick. This may be because carbohydrate has taken over the villain role, but also because of the real benefits of fats.

Reasons we need fats

- To absorb vitamins. Vitamins A, D, E and K can only be absorbed when we have fats in our diet. So, if we are avoiding fats or following a low-fat diet, then we can actually be doing the opposite by causing deficiencies.
- To maintain brain function. The brain is the fattiest organ of the body and is made up of 60% fat. To keep it functioning, we need to ensure we include essential fatty acids in our diet as our bodies cannot produce these. Fats are vital for brain development and structure, and have the important job of sending messages to your body.
- To keep our skin, hair and nails healthy.
- To slow down digestion, meaning you feel fuller for longer.
- To make food taste good! Compare the taste of a normal yoghurt and a low-fat version – which one tastes better and which one makes you feel more satisfied?

You might be thinking or even worrying that fats clog arteries and cause heart disease. There has been recent debate around the longstanding advice that fats should be avoided because of their detrimental impact on heart health. However, fats are actually important for the health of your heart.

Where do we get fats from?

- Oils
- Butter and margarine
- Mayonnaise and salad cream
- Oil-based salad dressings
- Avocados
- Nuts and seeds

We now know that no food group should be demonised, some fat is good for you, and it is important to include it in your diet.

FRUIT AND VEGETABLES

Although fruit and vegetables contain some carbohydrate, they do not contain enough for them to be counted as your main carbohydrate source, and so really shouldn't replace other carbohydrates on your plate.

"We now know that no food group should be demonised, some fat is good for you, and it is important to include it in your diet."

Fruit and vegetables are an essential part of balanced eating because they contain many of those micronutrients our body needs, as well as antioxidants for cell health, and fibre for a healthy digestive system. Because of this, fruit and vegetables are accepted as the "healthy" food to eat, and health campaigns have tried to get us all to eat more. But is more always better?

In an attempt to be healthier, there is nothing wrong with trying to eat more fruit and vegetables, but when they start to replace other nutrients, that can become a problem. When you look at the balanced eating plate earlier in this chapter, you will see that fruit and vegetables make up one third of the plate. So when we try to add more, something has got to give. That usually means either the amount of carbohydrate or protein gets smaller or is replaced altogether.

So, to get what you need, aim for your five a day by including one third of a plate of fruit and/or vegetables at your meals and as part of your snacks.

MICRONUTRIENTS

Rather than go through the benefits of each micronutrient and get bogged down with a lot of information, we will touch below on a couple of nutrients that we often see people excluding.

CALCIUM
Why do we need calcium?

Think of your bones as a "bank" where you "deposit" and "withdraw" bone tissue. During your childhood and teenage years, new bone is added (or deposited) to the skeleton faster than old bone is removed (or withdrawn). As a result, your bones become larger, heavier and denser. As you age, the reverse occurs; therefore it is important to ensure that the breakdown of bone is reduced as much as possible.

We are all aware that calcium is vital for our bones and teeth, and that is because 99% of our calcium is stored there and is important for bone integrity and strength. The final 1% is circulating in your blood. This 1% needs to stay topped up, because it is important for muscle contraction, including that of our heart. What does this mean? Simply put, if we don't get enough calcium from our diet to keep the calcium in our blood topped up, then our body starts to leech out calcium from our bones and teeth, to ensure our heart can continue to pump. This results in weaker bones, leading to osteopaenia (thinning of bone) and, if not rectified, osteoporosis, where bone becomes brittle and fragile, putting us at greater risk of fractures.

Where do we get calcium from?

- Dairy products, e.g. milk, yoghurt, cheese, custard
- Fish containing edible soft bones, e.g. canned pilchards, sardines
- Soya products, e.g. soya milk, soya yoghurt, tofu
- Cereal products, e.g. breakfast cereal and bread (as they tend to be fortified with calcium)
- Green leafy vegetables, e.g. spinach, broccoli, cabbage, kale, seaweed
- Pulses
- Sesame seeds
- Tap water in hard-water areas

Dairy foods have the best bioavailability for calcium, meaning we absorb more of the calcium contained within them than other foods. The others may have a high calcium content, but the bioavailability of that calcium is poorer, so we will not absorb a lot of it.

What can affect calcium absorption?

It is important to include vitamin D in your diet, as this plays an important role in calcium absorption. Vitamin D is made by the body through the action of sunlight on the skin, and is also found in foods such as mackerel, sardines, eggs, margarine and dairy products. This is why dairy has the best bioavailability of calcium, because these products contain calcium, vitamin D and phosphate – all of which increase absorption.

Plant foods have a lower bioavailability of calcium, even though their calcium content may be high. This is because they contain phytates and/or oxalates that bind to calcium and decrease calcium absorption. Therefore, if for some reason you are not eating dairy products, having a wide range of the other calcium-containing foods from the list will be more important.

If you drink a lot of tea and coffee, or eat a very high-protein diet or lots of salty food, this can also affect the absorption of calcium and can increase calcium loss from the body.

How do we get enough calcium?

The easiest way to get your calcium is through eating and drinking dairy products, e.g. a glass of milk, an individual pot of yoghurt or a slice of cheese. However, if you are not able to have dairy, then good alternatives can be soya milk and yoghurt, adding beans and pulses, choosing foods that are fortified with calcium, and sprinkling sesame seeds on your meal.

IRON

Why do we need iron?

Most of the iron found in the body is in haemoglobin. Haemoglobin is the protein in red blood cells that carry oxygen around the body and to the body's tissues. So, if we become iron deficient and develop iron deficiency anaemia, which occurs when your body doesn't have enough iron to produce haemoglobin. This results in tiredness and fatigue, pale skin, shortness of breath, heart palpitations and an increased risk of illness and infection.

Where do we get iron from?

- Red meat, e.g. beef, lamb, pork
- White meat, e.g. chicken, fish, seafood
- Liver
- Eggs
- Beans
- Nuts
- Dried fruit, such as dried apricots
- Wholegrains, such as brown rice
- Fortified breakfast cereals
- Soya products
- Most dark green leafy vegetables, e.g. spinach, kale

What we need to be aware of is that there are two different kinds of iron:

1. Haem iron – found in animal products
2. Non-haem iron – found in plant-based foods

Haem iron is easily absorbed by the body, whereas non-haem iron is not so easily absorbed. So, people who eat animal products can usually get enough iron from a balanced diet. However, if you are following a plant-based diet, it takes more effort and dedication to get adequate amounts of iron from food. You will need to eat twice as much iron-containing food as others who are eating animal products.

What can affect iron absorption?

As with calcium, there are several things that can affect iron absorption. Plants are only a non-haem source of iron, which as we've learned is harder for your body to absorb. Plant sources also contain phytates, which can hinder absorption. So, although spinach is famous for being a food high in iron, because it contains non-haem iron and phytates, we need to eat a lot of it to get our iron needs, and we need to help it along the way even then. To assist with absorption from non-haem iron sources, you can combine foods high in vitamin C in the same meal, like a glass of orange juice, citrus fruits, berries, peppers or potatoes. Likewise, it is also recommended that you try not to drink tea and coffee at the same time as food that contains non-haem iron, as the polyphenols within them can hinder absorption.

How do we get enough iron?

For those who eat animal products, you shouldn't have too much trouble getting enough iron into your body. Trying to ensure you eat a variety, including red meat and white meat, will be helpful. If you are following a plant-based diet, then you will need to make sure you are consuming beans and pulses, nuts and green leafy vegetables, and try to add a glass of orange juice to your meal. Also choosing foods that are fortified in iron, like some breakfast cereals, can be helpful.

Now we know what it is your body needs, let's explore why reducing or restricting our intake of these foods can be detrimental to our health.

CHAPTER 3

THE EFFECTS OF DIETING... AND WHY IT DOESN'T WORK

People often underestimate the impact dieting has on them. Although some people are intentionally trying to restrict their intake, others might believe they don't really need much food.

This is a myth.

About two-thirds of your daily energy requirements are for the essential functions in your body just to keep you alive. To keep your heart pumping, lungs inflating, kidneys filtering, blood circulating, brain neurons firing. And that's if you were comatose in bed, not moving a muscle. All the while, your body is doing some really hard work. Add to that the energy it takes to digest and absorb your food, for your immune system to keep you from getting sick or helping you recover from illness, for your body to constantly grow and repair itself, to produce testosterone or oestrogen/progesterone (and having a regular period), as well as your normal daily activity. And we haven't even counted any exercise yet!

So, what happens when we restrict our intake of food? Well, something has got to give. The body will react and start to prioritise: what non-essential functions can it feasibly stop expending energy on, so it can focus on your basic survival needs? Common reactions to dieting therefore include:

- Reduction in sex drive
- Tiredness and fatigue
- Deterioration of quality of skin, hair and nails
- Feeling cold

All of these occur because our body is trying to conserve energy for vital functions. But what if this is occurring and we still restrict even further, or we're forcing our body to expend more energy by exercising? Well, our body has to work even harder to conserve energy, so it will try to slow *everything* down. That means:

- Your heart rate slows down
- Your blood pressure drops
- Your digestive system slows down, which means you feel more bloated, constipated or have more abdominal discomfort than before. This is called "delayed gastric emptying"
- Your brain slows down, leading to difficulty concentrating, problem-solving and thinking in general
- Menstruation stops in women or you have irregular periods
- Your metabolism slows down

THE MINNESOTA EXPERIMENT

One of the best examples of how dieting can really affect us is the Minnesota Experiment.[3] Back in the 1940s, Ancel Keys led a study for which he recruited physically and psychologically healthy 20–30-year-old men who were conscientious war objectors. For the study, the men were "starved" by having their food intake cut in half. They were then observed to see what changes occurred. Interestingly, these men experienced almost all of the symptoms that are commonly experienced in those with a restrictive eating disorder. They included:

---

[3]   Keys, A., Brozek, J., Henschel, A., Mickelsen, O., Taylor, H.L. (1950). *The Biology of Human Starvation*. University of Minnesota Press: Minneapolis, MN, US.

Physical changes:
- Decreased need for sleep
- Dizziness and headaches
- Hypersensitivity to noise and light
- Reduced strength (even after a few days)
- Oedema (swelling)
- Tiredness
- Pain when sitting due to lack of body fat
- Feeling cold – particularly in hands and feet
- Slowing of metabolism
- Slowing of heart rate
- A 10% drop in blood volume
- A shrink in heart size
- Parasthesia (tingling) in hands and feet
- Gastrointestinal discomfort and constipation
- Hair loss

Cognitive changes:
- Impaired perception (despite weight loss, the men did not perceive themselves as excessively skinny; they actually thought everyone else looked too fat – more on this very common perception problem later)
- Increased preoccupation with food
- Impaired concentration and alertness
- Difficulties with comprehension and judgement

Behavioural changes:
- Obsessive food and eating behaviours – talking, reading and dreaming about it, and collecting cooking items; also an increase in hoarding
- Episodes of bingeing and purging
- An increase in time spent planning food
- Delaying their eating and taking up to two hours to eat a meal

- Eating in a ritualised way – in silence and with total attention to eating
- A huge increase in the use of salt and spices
- Eating up to 40 packs of gum and drinking 15 coffees per day.

Emotional changes:
- Increased episodes of depression
- Increased anxiety
- Increased levels of apathy
- An increase in irritability and outbursts of anger
- Neglect of hygiene

Social and sexual changes:
- Increased social withdrawal and isolation
- Decreased humour and companionship
- Impaired libido

Remember, these men were physically and psychologically healthy prior to participating in this study, and yet the lack of adequate calories caused a number of detrimental effects on their mind, body and behaviour. Are we really surprised, therefore, when we see these same symptoms occurring in people who restrict their food intake?

The good news is, when the men's food intake increased again and they started to gain weight, the symptoms improved. Some symptoms improved more quickly than others, but they found that they *only* started to improve when they were given more food than their *pre-experiment* amounts. This allowed for re-nourishment and weight restoration. Their weight initially fluctuated, but after about a year it settled at around their pre-experiment weight (or within their normal range).

Perhaps have a look at the above information and think about whether you are experiencing any of these issues. Many people identify with at least a few of these symptoms.

WHY DIETING DOESN'T WORK: DEPRIVATION

As we have mentioned earlier, diets do not have a high success rate. Despite this, there are hundreds out there and people constantly go back and try new ones in an effort to control their weight.

If a doctor were to give you medication for an illness, but it only had a small chance of working and had a whole list of side effects, would you take it? Would you keep going back for more when it didn't work? Would you blame *yourself* when it didn't work? Would your doctor keep insisting that you need to try it again?

"Why is it that dieting doesn't work? This can be summed up in one word: deprivation."

If dieting worked, there would be just one diet that everyone followed instead of the many that are out there.

So, why is it that dieting doesn't work? This can be summed up in one word: deprivation.

Deprivation can be physical or psychological. When you consistently do not eat enough, your body will crave energy because you are forcing it into a negative energy balance, which it doesn't like. Ever tried to restrict your food intake to lose weight, only to "fall off the wagon" and eat anything (or everything) you find in the cupboard because you get too hungry? This is because food is the fuel we need to survive. When running low, our body will drive us to eat so that we have enough energy for our vital functions, to keep us generally healthy and, well, alive!

DEPRIVATION OF NUTRITION

As we've spoken about already, when we don't eat enough, our body begins to prioritise our vital functions with the energy it does get. As a part of this process, our metabolism slows down – which is not a good thing. Despite eating very little, our weight plateaus and if, in an effort to keep losing weight, we try to restrict even more, this only makes our metabolism slow down further.

When we are not giving our body sufficient energy, it looks for other available sources and will start to break down our reserves. It will use the carbohydrate stores in our muscle and liver first, because they are the best source of available energy, and then move on to break down our body fat and skeletal muscle. We cannot tell our body to break down *only* fat, so it breaks down both, and we really don't want to lose muscle. Muscle and our metabolism, i.e. the rate at which we convert food into energy, are closely related: losing muscle means our metabolism slows down. Remember that our organs are also muscles, and these too may be broken down and damaged in our body's attempt to get more energy.

"The answer is not just to eat *more*, but to eat more consistently."

So, what's the answer to help speed up our metabolism? Eat more! The body needs to feel reassured that it will consistently get enough energy to fuel those vital functions, before it can relax. It needs to know it will always have enough energy so that it does not need to draw on its own reserves. So, the answer is not just to eat *more*, but to eat more *consistently*.

DEPRIVATION OF FOOD TYPES

Deprivation can also involve certain types of food. Have you ever said to yourself, "I'm never going to eat chocolate or crisps again", and then, although you may resist at first, the craving gets so intense that you end up eating a whole family-size bar/

pack? Yep, that's deprivation right there. You may be eating enough throughout the day, but you are not allowing yourself to eat the foods you *want*. This gives them a "special" and powerful status in your mind, which they don't need to have.

If we are deprived because we have taboo foods, then we need to make peace with food and start giving ourselves permission to eat these foods again, whenever we want, and as part of a healthy balanced lifestyle (as explained in Chapter 2).

"LAST SUPPER" EATING

Deprivation can also trigger "Last Supper" eating. Say, for example, you have put chocolate biscuits on your "forbidden foods" list. On the occasions you eat a chocolate biscuit, you then push the "Sod it" or "I give up" button, thinking, "I've messed up now and so I may as well eat the whole pack..." You may even think that you need to "get rid of" the food from the house by eating it all. All this probably would not have happened if chocolate biscuits were allowed in the first place.

SET POINT THEORY

There is yet another way that we deprive ourselves: by depriving our body of its natural weight and shape. Just like we are born with a predetermined height, we are also born with a predetermined weight range. This is called our *set point range*. Just like our height, our weight can be influenced by environment, e.g. if we have suffered neglect and poor nutrition. However, genetics is the main influencing factor on our weight.

If we diet and lose weight, our body tries its hardest to regulate our weight and get it back to our set point range. It does this by sending out hunger signals, increasing the number of thoughts and obsessions around food, and slowing down our metabolism. If we ignore these signals, our body just works even harder to do this. Think of your set point range as a thermostat in your house. If you set the temperature to 20 degrees, you know that if the temperature falls below that, the heating will kick in and get your house back up to the temperature on the thermostat. You can try to control the temperature yourself by opening a window to let cool air in, but if you do, the heating will only come on with more force in order to get the house back up to 20 degrees. The same thing happens with our bodies. It happens because our set point is the weight range at which we are most healthy and function at our best.

So, can we control or dictate our set point? Unfortunately not. It doesn't matter how hard we try, our set point will not change. The exception to this is, if you diet all the time, your set point can actually shift *upwards*. This is why people who chronically diet end up yo-yoing in weight and may ultimately gain weight over time.

The myths that we can choose to lose weight below our natural range and that we can diet healthily, are so damaging. We cannot change our genetics. To have a better relationship with food and our body, we need to work on acceptance of the body we naturally have.

POODLE SCIENCE

There is a really cool three-minute YouTube clip called "Poodle Science,"[4] which explains how our body weight and shape is mainly governed by our genes and how it does not define our health. Why not take a few minutes to watch it now?

---

[4]   Association for Size Diversity and Health (ASDAH) (2015). *Poodle Science*. [Online video] Available at: www.youtube.com/watch?v=H89QQfXtc-k [Accessed 30 July 2020].

HUNGER HORMONES

Our hormones are critical to helping our bodies fight deprivation.

Adults who eat intuitively can maintain their weight over time without much effort, just by listening to their internal cues. We have two hormones that govern our appetite to thank for that: ghrelin and leptin. Ghrelin is a fast-acting hormone that *stimulates* our appetite, while leptin is the slower-acting hormone that *suppresses* appetite. These hormones work together to signal to us our body's needs and ensure we are consistently nourished.

When our stomach is empty, ghrelin, the appetite-stimulating hormone, is secreted and signals to our brain that we are hungry. As you can imagine, if we have been fasting, delaying our eating or restricting our intake, higher levels of ghrelin will be released. Once we eat, ghrelin secretion is suppressed. However, for chronic dieters, ghrelin levels may stay high, because of the constant state of hunger they are in as a result of not feeding themselves enough. Makes sense, doesn't it? Remember, this is our body's mechanism for survival that ensures we are nourished and not in a state of starvation. It's no wonder that when we diet, the hunger signals to our brain intensify. The more we restrict, the more ghrelin is produced. The longer we put our bodies under that stress, the more forcefully and insistently our body will try to signal to us that it needs more food.

> "The longer we put our bodies under that stress, the more forcefully and insistently our body will try to signal to us that it needs more food."

Leptin, the appetite-suppressing hormone, is released into the circulatory system by the adipose (fat) tissues and travels to the brain to give it information about the body's energy stores. When the body has more fat stores, it causes an increase in leptin levels. This results in a reduction in appetite, and an increase in energy expenditure to maintain the amount of body fat stores.

Conversely, when someone diets or loses weight, leptin levels drop, resulting in increased appetite and food intake, and decreased energy expenditure (or metabolism).

Leptin also signals to the brain that we are full and satisfied with what we have eaten. If someone diets and/or loses weight, leptin is suppressed, and the feeling of fullness and satisfaction is often not felt. This is a reason that many people who diet often complain of just never feeling full, and why, in the long run, dieting doesn't work.

So, what about cravings? Well, there is a neurotransmitter called neuropeptide-Y that *really* doesn't like us starving ourselves. It signals in the brain that we are hungry. And not just any old hunger – hunger for carbohydrates specifically. Neuropeptide-Y increases the motivation and urgency to eat, and results in us needing to eat more to get that feeling of fullness and satisfaction. So it's no wonder that when we diet or restrict our food intake, we specifically crave bread, crisps, biscuits or cake, and that it often feels as if, if we don't eat it right now, we will not survive. So, when we reach for those foods, it's because neuropeptide-Y is screaming at us, and it's not surprising that not only do we eat them like our life depends on it (and it kind of does!), but that we eat much more than we would if we hadn't been restricting or dieting.

Now that we have looked at the impact of dieting and the costs of deprivation on our physical and psychological health, let's consider some other behaviours people use to try to control their eating, feelings or body.

CHAPTER 4

WHY COMPENSATORY BEHAVIOURS DON'T WORK

After eating, some people find themselves searching for a strategy to counteract fullness, prevent weight gain, or rid themselves of feelings such as guilt, regret or shame. These are sometimes known as compensatory behaviours because they are often motivated by an attempt to compensate for eating in order to avoid feared consequences. With these hopes in mind, people might misuse laxatives, take diet pills, make themselves vomit, obsessively exercise, or return back to an extreme diet.

Compensatory behaviours can be some of the most shocking elements of eating problems. We commonly find that people realise there is a problem when they find themselves trying things like vomiting or buying diet pills online. These behaviours tend to be very private, given the level of guilt and embarrassment people often feel about them. They are also an aspect of an eating problem that others find most difficult to understand. Everything we do as human beings is driven by an underlying need, and in the instance of compensatory behaviours, this is usually to feel in control of our bodies or eating. The fact that people turn to these extreme behaviours is evidence of the strength of the desire to control eating.

If this is you, we understand that the pattern could be so entrenched by now or feel so overwhelming that making change might seem difficult. Even so, let's spend some time understanding these behaviours and their consequences in more detail, to help you move forward.

THE CYCLES OF COMPENSATION

Most of the time, people who engage in these behaviours want to stop but find it incredibly hard. So what keeps these behaviours going? Let's take some time to explore this together.

1. YOUR BELIEF ABOUT THE EFFECTIVENESS OF THESE BEHAVIOURS

Most people engage in these behaviours, and continue to do so, because they believe they help them lose weight. Often, when people start to eat, they might give themselves "permission" for bingeing by thinking they will "just use a compensatory behaviour" after. This permissive thought will lead to a greater urge later to follow through with the compensatory behaviour. However, vomiting, diet pills and laxatives *aren't very effective* in counteracting calorie intake, so aren't going to help you meet the goal anyway (more on this later).

2. THE BEHAVIOURS EMOTIONALLY REINFORCE THE EATING PROBLEM

In the short term, these behaviours make you feel positive feelings. For example, you might momentarily feel relief after laxative use or proud of your extreme exercise. In the long term, however, you end up feeling bad again. Perhaps you get tired, can't continue the exercise at the rate you were previously achieving, and feel like you've failed. Or maybe after vomiting or using laxatives you feel a sense of disgust, or fear that these behaviours have become uncontrollable. These unpleasant feelings might then trigger further eating problems, for example bingeing or dieting. Any which way, the cycle of problematic eating and compensation continues and you feel stuck.

3. THE PHYSICAL CONSEQUENCES CAN KEEP THE URGE TO USE THE BEHAVIOURS GOING

Your body physically adjusts as you are using these behaviours. For example, if you use laxatives and feel better immediately, before long you will become more sensitive to the feeling of being full and may even become constipated. It may then take more laxatives to get the desired effect, and you might ultimately become reliant on them or feel out of control. If you have a tendency to restrict your food intake, you might feel full and uncomfortable when you eat so you delay your next meal and then fast for a long period of time after. This means that when you do eat, you're more likely to feel uncomfortably full again (more on this below).

THE PHYSICAL EFFECTS OF COMPENSATORY BEHAVIOURS

LAXATIVES

Laxatives are ineffective for weight loss and have a detrimental impact. People start using laxatives in the short term to relieve constipation. Some laxatives work by irritating the large bowel so that the contents are expelled more quickly. While the speed of this prevents vital minerals and water being reabsorbed into your body, it *does not* reduce calorie intake (because calories have already been absorbed in the small intestine).

People might try laxatives in an effort to feel "empty" or lighter, achieve a flat stomach, or in the pursuit of weight loss. However, any change in weight is only a temporary result of water loss. This is not permanent. This water loss or dehydration can be dangerous as you can drastically reduce and disrupt the electrolytes in your body, in particular potassium. This can have serious health effects, such as abnormal heart rhythms which can lead to heart attacks.

Overuse of laxatives can also cause the bowel to become lazy, making it much harder to go to the toilet naturally. Excessive straining when going to the toilet becomes common. This can cause bleeding due to a blood vessel in the bowel becoming fragile, or in extreme cases even a rectal prolapse.

SIDE EFFECTS OF LAXATIVE MISUSE

- Depletion of water and vital minerals in your body
- Low potassium, which can trigger cardiac problems
- Low electrolyte levels, which can cause muscle weakness, confusion and convulsions
- Dehydration, leading to kidney problems/failure or urinary tract infections (UTIs)
- Painful cramps, chronic constipation and bloating
- Ulcers (due to diarrhoea)
- Rectal bleeding
- Loss of muscle tone in the bowel
- Damage to the muscles in your bowel, causing incontinence (with prolonged use)

VOMITING

Sometimes people make themselves vomit in an attempt to lose weight or prevent weight gain, or in a response to emotional triggers. People believe they are getting rid of all the calories they've eaten by vomiting. However, like laxatives, vomiting is very ineffective and has a number of physical side effects.

More than half of calories consumed are retained in the body after vomiting. So how does it all work? First, some calories have already been absorbed in the mouth before the food even reaches the stomach. Second, while some food is pushed out of the mouth during vomiting, approximately half is pushed further down the gastrointestinal tract and into the small intestine. Once it is in the small intestine, it cannot be purged.

Some people judge what they have vomited by looking out for food "markers" in an attempt to confirm what they have actually purged, thinking that the first food they ate will be the last food to come out. However, this strategy does not work as the stomach mixes food up in a "washing-machine" action, so what you have eaten at the beginning could be anywhere in the stomach when you vomit.

After eating, the body produces insulin to be able to utilise the sugar it expects to absorb from the food. Although vomiting gets rid of some food, insulin is still released and levels remain high. This results in low blood-sugar level, which then sends a signal to the brain to say you are hungry and need to eat. This leads to craving food and possibly another binge episode.

SIDE EFFECTS OF VOMITING

- Dehydration due to fluid loss. This in turn can result in:
  - feeling weak, light-headed and faint
  - frequent urinary tract infections (short term)
  - kidney damage (long term)
- The salivary glands in the face swell up, giving a puffy appearance or more rounded face
- The mouth and throat can become sore, causing a hoarse voice or infections
- The oesophagus can become sore, inflamed, or bleed
- Distension of the stomach and oesophagus (ruptures can also occur, which are rare but potentially fatal)
- Electrolyte imbalance. When you vomit, you lose electrolytes from your body, which affects nerve and muscle function. This can cause muscle weakness/spasms, convulsions and potentially fatal problems with the rhythm and function of the heart
- Over time, damage to the muscles at the top of the stomach which are designed to keep food in, leading to reflux and heartburn

- Over time, dental problems due to stomach acid eroding the enamel on your teeth, causing cavities, sensitivity and pain

DIET PILLS

Diet pills can come in many different forms, contain different ingredients and cause different side effects. They usually claim to help burn fat, stop fat absorption by the body, reduce appetite, or boost metabolism. But they usually don't deliver what they promise and they can be really dangerous.

Diet pills are not often regulated, so they can claim to have all sorts of benefits that are unfounded. They can also contain substances that have been banned because of their harmful effects. Human studies showing any actual effect on weight loss are rare when it comes to diet pills. If some effect has been shown, it is short term and usually accompanied by some nasty side effects.

In the best-case scenario, diet pills will have no effect; essentially performing the role of a placebo and leaving you out of pocket. In the worst-case scenario, they can cause some very serious damage.

SIDE EFFECTS OF DIET-PILL USE

- As diet pills often contain high doses of caffeine, they can often cause headaches, tremors, diarrhoea, rapid heart rate, anxiety and reduced sleep
- Some diet pills claim to reduce fat absorption, but will also cause abdominal pain, flatulence, diarrhoea or incontinence, and nutrient deficiencies
- Because some diet pills have substances that have been banned or are unknown, they can cause a variety of different side effects ranging from nausea, bleeding, blurred vision, heart problems, to damage to vital organs, and death

OBSESSIVE EXERCISE

A healthy amount of activity is necessary to keep our body and mind happy and healthy. When exercise tips into being driven, punishing or overly rigid or excessive, however, it has become a problem. Driven or obsessive exercise is another strategy people use to manage the feared consequences or difficult feelings related to eating. If this is you, exercise might preoccupy your thoughts and you might hold the view that you can only eat in a certain way if you work out afterwards. And if you don't exercise, you might be left with feelings of guilt or self-loathing and associated negative thoughts. In obsessive exercise, there is very little pleasure anymore. Enjoyment is replaced with gruelling, and often solitary, regimes. As such, your exercise regime is not only preoccupying your mind, but your daily schedule, and is actually interfering with your life. If you are noticing huge amounts of guilt or anxiety related to exercise, have a think about the impact of your exercise on your mental wellbeing.

What might indicate that I have a problem with obsessive exercise?

- You are rigid with your exercise routine
- You prioritise exercise over other areas of your life
- You eat less if you can't exercise
- You exercise even if you are injured or unwell
- You exercise to change your weight and shape rather than for enjoyment
- If you can't exercise it "ruins your day"

SIDE EFFECTS OF EXCESSIVE EXERCISE

- Bone damage and increased stress fractures
- Cardiac problems
- Semi-starvation effects if you are not eating sufficiently including anxiety and obsessive behaviour (see "Extreme Dieting")
- The "Female Athlete Triad". This is a condition in which the person has low energy availability because they are not eating enough and exercising too much, resulting in a negative energy balance. It causes menstrual dysfunction and low bone density. This condition is not only seen in people with eating problems
- "Relative Energy Deficiency in Sport" (REDS). This is a condition comprising a lowering of hormone levels, a deterioration in bone density leading to fractures and injury, a lowering of metabolism, and a deterioration in mental health

EXTREME DIETING

Extreme dieting and fasting might also be used as a means of attempted compensating. We have already talked about the problems with dieting, but, put simply, extreme dieting or restriction leads to the state of semi-starvation. This causes both physical and psychological changes that can make eating more difficult.

One common effect of extreme dieting, as already mentioned, is "delayed gastric emptying" (the slowing down of food moving through the digestive system) because of loss of stomach muscle tone and loss of energy. This means it takes a lot longer for food to pass through to your small intestine. As the food sits longer in your stomach, you are likely to experience bloating, nausea, early satiety (getting full quite quickly after eating), pain/discomfort and constipation. Although it will feel uncomfortable, the only way to get your digestive system working properly again is to eat more and accept that you will feel uncomfortable, but that it will pass over time – you just need to persist with it.

> "Being hungry, or feeling stressed, are both precursors to binge eating."

As you now know, putting your body into a state of semi-starvation can have some serious side effects. It can also set you up to react to the psychological and physical deprivation by seeking out food in a more out-of-control way. Being hungry, or feeling stressed, are both precursors to binge eating.

We have explored a range of problems people face in relation to their eating. Some might be relevant to you, and some not. It's time now to think about how the problems we have outlined apply to you and how you can use this information in order to move forward. Join us in thinking about your readiness to make change.

PART II

FIRST STEPS

CHAPTER 5

TIME TO CHANGE?

The fact that you have picked this book up suggests that you are interested in making changes to your eating. This is a great first step. But we know that being motivated to change our behaviour and *staying* motivated is easier said than done. Let's face it, changing our behaviour is hard.

The Stages of Change Model, developed by Prochaska and DiClemente, is a useful model when thinking about motivation to change our behaviour. They propose that there are five key stages to making and maintaining change:

- Pre-contemplation – believing there is no problem and no need for change
- Contemplation – realising there is a problem and having thoughts about how life could be different if you make change
- Preparation – deciding to change and making plans about how to do so
- Action – actively making steps to change
- Maintenance – keeping the new behaviour going

Have a look at these five stages, and think where you might be. Are you contemplating change, or already making changes to your eating behaviour? Are you preparing to make changes soon, but not quite there yet?

Knowing which stage of change you are at will help you figure out what you need at this point in your journey. You might move between these stages – and that is okay. Indeed, we imagine that if you have picked up this book, you might find yourself moving between the pre-contemplation and contemplation stages of change. If this is you, it is a good idea to think honestly about how much you want to change. It is really normal to feel in two minds about change. Feeling pressured to change before you are ready is unlikely to create lasting change, so we think the best first step is to be honest with yourself. This involves taking a close look at the impact of your eating problem and how it affects your life. The exercises that follow are designed to help with this.

> "It is really normal to feel in two minds about change."

PROS AND CONS

One way to think about your readiness to change is to construct a pros and cons list. These can be helpful in life when we need to make a decision about anything. Often the ideas are already floating around in our head, but it is helpful to put these down on paper.

EXERCISE: PROS AND CONS

Make a list of all of the aspects of your current eating behaviour that you might consider a "pro" (i.e. beneficial to you) and then beside that make another list of the aspects of your eating that are a "con" (i.e. not beneficial). Try to think about all aspects of your life, for example: relationships, physical health, financial, psychological health, work/education and life enjoyment.

When you are considering a pros and cons list, hold in mind the following:

1. ***Don't forget to think about short- and long-term pros and cons.*** As human beings we focus more on the immediate consequences and can lose track of our long-term goals. It might feel as if there are quite a few advantages to your eating behaviour in the short term; however, in the long term it's a different story. In Clare's list (shown below), she writes that her eating problems give her some feelings of control in the short term, but in the long term make her feel unhappy. She also realised that using her eating as a way of managing stress was actually a disadvantage to her in the long term.

2. ***Have a read of the information in this book about the consequences of particular eating problems.*** Some of this is likely to be relevant for a thorough pros and cons list. For example, Chapters 3 and 4 highlight some of the short- and long-term physical and psychological effects on your mind and body of undereating, or using compensatory behaviours.

Remember Clare, from the introduction? This would be her list:

PROS OF MY EATING BEHAVIOUR	CONS OF MY EATING BEHAVIOUR
It helps me feel in control	I'm obsessed with food
It makes my weight stay low	I can't eat out with my friends
It gives me a sense of achievement	I'm tired all the time
People compliment me	My boyfriend gets frustrated with me
It helps me feel less stressed	I feel like I'm failing all the time

Now you have a go:

PROS	CONS

Once you've completed your list, think about whether you have written down *facts*. Or, instead, are they feelings or fears and not necessarily representative of reality? Often we believe our thoughts and feelings are 100% accurate simply because they feel so true to us. For example, Clare thought that her eating behaviour helped manage her weight, but this was actually a fear rather than a reality, given what you now know about the effectiveness of dieting.

Have a think, too, about whether some of your pros are about needs that you *currently* meet via your eating behaviour, but that could be met another way. For example, Clare found that restricting her eating gave her a sense of achievement. Although this certainly *feels* like a pro to Clare, there are actually other (less fleeting) ways of getting that sense of achievement, such as learning a new hobby or skill. Go through your pros and cons list now and circle anything that you think is a need that could potentially be met in another way that does not come with the same consequences.

VALUES

Having a focus on your eating and your body can take up a lot of time and energy. Sometimes it preoccupies your mind so much that it means other things that are important to you are neglected. In order to think about your eating and your body in the wider context of your life, it is helpful to consider your values.

Values are the things that are important to us as individuals. They give us direction, meaning and purpose. Values are different to goals, which are specific and measurable. Values are more like a guide that we constantly work towards. If we imagine the recovery journey as being a trail away from your eating difficulties and towards wellness, then your values are like a compass, providing direction. There will be obstacles along the journey as well as smoother terrain, but your values will help you stay on track.

EXERCISE: VALUES

Take some time to think about your values. Not what you think they *should* be, or what your siblings'/parents'/partner's values are, but the things that *you* value. We all value different things in life.

Here is Chris's list:

MY VALUES

Being a good boyfriend	Being caring
Being hardworking	Learning
Being respected	Success
Being honest	Fun

Now it's your turn. What do you value in life?

Now look at your list and ask yourself the following questions:

- How much is my eating behaviour and relationship with food helping me move towards or away from these values?
- What needs to change in order for my eating behaviour to be more in line with my values?

In Chris's case, he could see that his eating problems were in fact pulling him away from his values. They brought on strong feelings of shame, which led to secrecy, and this stopped him from having the honest and caring relationship he wanted with his partner. He was also caught sometimes so preoccupied with food that it stopped him focusing on his relationship, which upset him. He also noticed that his eating was interfering with his focus at work. When he realised this, Chris tried to shift his focus onto that which was truly important to him and devoted his time and energy to the things that really mattered, such as scheduling some fun activities with his partner.

Reminding ourselves of our values can be a helpful way to stay focused on what is important – in this case, our recovery!

IMAGINE YOUR FUTURE

While we are exploring change, it is also helpful to think about what your life will look like in the future.

EXERCISE: YOUR FUTURE SELF

Set some time aside to think about the life you want to live in one year's time, as well as five years' time. What do you want to be doing on a daily basis? Where do you want to live? Who will you be spending time with? Are you happy in this life? How are your relationships? How is your health?

Here's what Clare thought about:

MY FUTURE SELF

1 year's time:

Living in my hometown	Working
In a stable relationship	Going out to the pub or for walks in the park

5 years' time:

Trying to have a child	In a secure relationship
Got a promotion	Have a puppy
Travelled to South America	Taken regular summer holiday with friends

Don't worry if your ideas currently feel out of reach. Have some fun thinking about your future. Some people find this task a bit difficult, but allowing yourself to imagine what your future could look like is what will help motivate you.

Once you've imagined your life in one as well as five years' time, ask yourself: where does my eating problem fit in with this future? Do I still have eating problems when I'm imagining my future self?

When Clare reflected on this, she realised that in this future she didn't imagine being so preoccupied with eating and her body. She imagined herself having a better relationship with food. She imagined being able to eat flexibly on summer holidays, to go into restaurants that she wanted. She didn't see herself asking her boyfriend for reassurance about her eating, and her exercise regime wasn't as punishing. Overall, her imagined future self felt more content in her life. Clare reminded herself of this to help her stay motivated.

GOAL-SETTING

We hope that by looking into the future you are inspired to make changes to your eating. If so, have a think about what your future self thinks you, in the present, need to do to make a change right now.

Goals are important, as they will help you reach your final destination and commit to the changes you really want to make. Rather than your goal being "to have a better relationship with food" or "to improve my eating" (which are great aims), we encourage you to try to make it a bit more specific and to break it up into small, achievable targets. Remember that they should be measurable, so you can identify when each one has been completed.

EXERCISE: YOUR GOALS

Think about some measureable goals you would like to achieve in the next month. Here is a list of Clare's goals, as an example:
- Reduce weighing myself to only once a week
- To go out with my friends for dinner this Saturday
- To eat a food I have been avoiding, such as chocolate

Now, make your own list:

Keep revisiting these goals to check you are on the right path and living according to your values and the future life you want.

It might be a good idea to return to these exercises if you find your motivation wanes. This is a normal part of change and we encourage you to stay focused on the life you want. We believe you can do this!

It might also be a good idea to share your above reflections and goals for change with someone you trust, so they can help support you. More on this in the next chapter.

CHAPTER 6

FINDING SUPPORT

Overcoming your eating problems is no easy task. In our experience, many people want to make improvements to their eating, and feel extremely motivated, but still find it challenging. Often, people have tried many times before they can actually improve their relationship with food. Having a support network, or your own cheerleaders, can make a world of difference. Your support system is like a structure to prop things up for you if you're feeling vulnerable, and can be of great practical and emotional value. We like to think of our support as equivalent to the scaffolding on a house that is undergoing renovations. They give you stability when you feel fragile and might only need to support you in this way for a period of time.

"Your support system is like a structure to prop things up for you if you're feeling vulnerable, and can be of great practical and emotional value."

Have a think about the people in your support crew. It might include a person with whom you can share a meal that you have historically found challenging. Or there may be a family member who will sit with you if you feel driven to exercise or even vomit after eating. Your support crew can also remind you of your goals and values at times when you lose sight of these. They aren't necessarily people who will solve problems; they might simply be there for you when you need them to be.

Perhaps you haven't told anyone about your struggle. This is not unusual, as eating problems can feel very private. However, try to think now of the supportive people in your life and how they might be able to help cheerlead you to better eating patterns. Don't be afraid to be selective with this choice. Think about someone who will be respectful and considerate.

Have a look below at some of the potential qualities of a support person and consider those qualities that matter the most to you. Bear in mind that no one person can be all of these things for us at all times, so you should aim to find someone who generally has these qualities:

- Understanding of your eating problem
- Compassionate
- Encouraging
- Willing to listen to how you feel
- Willing to challenge you
- Able to eat with you
- Able to face eating challenges with you
- Able to spend time with you after eating

We would also like to encourage you to bring these qualities to yourself as you face your eating problem. We have often found that the people we work with are their own harshest critic. Ask yourself: do you bring this same supportive approach to yourself? Are you truly being part of your own support crew?

As mentioned, it may be that you feel very private about your eating issues, or perhaps even ashamed. You might worry that you will be judged, or have concerns about being a burden to others. These experiences and perceptions can create an obstacle to sharing your

"Are you truly being part of your own support crew?"

struggles with loved ones. We sometimes forget that other people have had their own difficulties in life. You never know when you will need to return the supporting favour! In our experience, having conversations about our struggles can actually bring us closer to others. You might be the person who enables others to speak up too. We have heard so many people talk about making the decision to share their feelings and vulnerabilities with great trepidation, only to find that their fear was unfounded.

As we mentioned earlier, if you think you need more support, please seek professional face-to-face input, especially if your eating problems are worsening and feel overwhelming. However, even with professional support, don't underestimate how helpful loved ones can be. We all need to have a support crew in life.

"Don't underestimate how helpful loved ones can be. We all need to have a support crew in life."

We have looked at how you can draw on support from others to help you on this journey of overcoming your eating problem. We look next at how you can also support yourself in making change by becoming more aware of your own eating and the associated thoughts and feelings.

CHAPTER 7

BECOMING AWARE

An important start to improving your relationship with food is understanding where the problem lies. This means being aware of what is going on around you, within you, and with your eating. One way to increase awareness is to keep a journal. We'll give you some guidance below on the most helpful way to do this for an eating problem. Keeping a journal will help you activate your inner detective by uncovering clues about what is driving your eating problems, so you know where to intervene. If you're tempted to skip this chapter (as, for many, reflecting on and writing about their eating problems feels like a bad idea), please read on and at least give it some thought.

Take the analogy of your eating problems being akin to a fire. When assessing the nature and impact of a blaze, firefighters

"Keeping a journal will help you activate your inner detective by uncovering clues about what is driving your eating problems, so you know where to intervene."

first would want to know: 1) the conditions that led to the fire starting (i.e. any existing vulnerabilities to eating problems) and 2) what ignited the specific fire (i.e. what the trigger for a specific eating behaviour was). And, of course, the task isn't just to observe a fire, but to put it out and prevent a repeat. So, to prevent future eating problem "fires" in our own lives, we first need to identify the conditions that brought us to this point, so we can make changes on this front, and then learn to notice when there is a spark igniting, so we can intervene before it gets out of control.

WHY KEEP A JOURNAL?

A journal has many helpful roles in overcoming an eating problem. Broadly, it helps you to notice your thoughts and feelings, and how situations are impacting you, and links these to your eating problems. More specifically:

1. Being aware of these factors is the starting point for change, as it gets you out of "autopilot".

Once you are out of autopilot, you will identify moments in your life at which you can decide to take a different path. The more aware you are of what's going on, the more opportunities you will have to step away from your eating problem.

Writing down what is happening at the time, will give you an opportunity to reflect later on, when you are feeling relaxed enough to think. You can then look through your journal with curiosity about what led you to the eating behaviour you are struggling with. For example, in the instance of Chris, he noticed his eating behaviour deteriorated at the times when his mood was flatter.

Noticing these patterns will help you feel a greater sense of understanding by enlightening you, rather than it all feeling like an impossible situation.

2. It is a chance to be compassionate and understanding towards yourself.

It is important not to use the journal in a punishing way. The purpose is not to use it to calorie count, obsess more or criticise yourself. Rather, the intention is to bring an approach of gentle curiosity in order to start the process of change. There are good reasons why you do the things you do, and why eating has become a problem. Try to remind yourself of that.

3. A journal can provide a much-needed reality check and a level of self-accountability.

We realise that for some this can feel difficult or even painful. One of the reasons eating problems thrive is because it can feel too difficult to address the problem and the reality of your eating problem is easier to avoid. Remember though, to bring that compassionate understanding to the reality check!

For some, it may be easier to write what you have eaten but more difficult to acknowledge what you were feeling. For others, being specific with what you have eaten can feel challenging enough. Either way, we encourage you to try your best to complete all aspects of the journaling process below, as this will help you to better understand any patterns or trends and, ultimately, will provide clues of where changes can be made.

GETTING STARTED

When journaling to help overcome an eating problem, it's helpful to work on increasing awareness of your thoughts and feelings, and your eating behaviours. You will want to record each of these things in order to find the links between them. If you can't notice your thoughts and feelings straight away, don't worry. We talk more about identifying these later on in this book. Right now, just focus on starting the process of becoming more aware. This means keeping a journal in which you routinely record:

- What is happening in your day
- What you are eating/drinking (see example for level of detail)
- Binges or out-of-control eating
- Compensatory behaviours, including:
  - Restricting or limiting the amount or type of food you eat
  - Vomiting

- ○ Laxative use
- ○ Diet-pill use
- Exercise – note how much and how driven this was
- What you are thinking
- What you are feeling

In order to get started, find a way that suits you to complete your journal – whether that is in a handwritten form, or on your phone. There are also some good apps out there, for example Recovery Record, which could be a helpful tool as it is designed for people with disordered eating and eating disorders. Whichever format you choose, we recommend you complete the journal "in the moment" as much as possible. This makes it easier to recall everything you have eaten as well as what the specific circumstances were at the time.

"Through journaling you can work on increasing awareness of your thoughts and feelings, and your eating behaviours."

We also recommend you record as much information as possible, to help with reflecting on a broad pattern later on. For example, record any mood fluctuations as you may not be aware at the time that these contribute to your eating behaviour, but when you reflect on a week's worth of journalling you can see a pattern of emotional eating. Also, record all your exercise, as you may not realise at the time that there is a problem, but when you look back you can see a pattern of obsessive or excessive exercise.

On the next page, there is an example of a structure you *could* use in your journal. This is what Suki might write:

DATE: 4 JANUARY 2020				
TIME	FOOD AND DRINK CONSUMED	WAS IT A BINGE?	CB*	WHAT WAS GOING ON? (THOUGHTS, FEELINGS, SITUATION)
7am	Black coffee One piece of toast with jam			Felt tired. Had to quickly eat something before the school run.
10am				At work. Felt hungry but thought "I'm not going to give in".
12pm	Half a bread roll Vegetable soup			I really tried to not have a whole bread roll because I had toast this morning. I still felt hungry but I need to pursue this diet if I want to lose weight.
3pm	Chocolate biscuit			I shouldn't have had that. Felt guilty. They were at the meeting though and I couldn't stop myself.
3.30pm			Run	I'm tired but I had to work off that biscuit and make sure that I ran for longer than yesterday.
5.30pm	7 fish fingers 3 slices of cheese Handful of oven fries 4 chocolate biscuits	Yes		Preparing my kids' dinner and was not planning on eating with them tonight. Stuff it. I already had a chocolate biscuit, so what's another? The day's ruined. I just couldn't stop myself.
8pm	Half a bowl of stir-fry			My husband asked why I wasn't eating much. I'm so ashamed. Tomorrow will be different. I'm going to do 2 classes at the gym back to back.
11.30pm	2 chocolate biscuits			Hungry again. Feel so greedy.

* Compensatory behaviours (include vomiting, diet pills, laxatives, obsessive exercise, restricting)

REFLECTING

When you have started completing your journal, set aside time every day or every few days to look back at the entries. Read them with open-minded curiosity, remembering to be compassionate to yourself in the process.

Some questions you might ask yourself as you go through your journal include:

- Did I eat regularly?
- Did I deprive myself in any way?
- Did I eat enough?
- Did I eat in a balanced way including all food groups during the day?
- Are there particular situations that are linked to problem eating behaviours?
- Are there particular emotions that are linked to the problematic eating?
- Are there particular thoughts that keep coming up?
- Was my exercise reasonable? Or driven/excessive/obsessive?

As you begin to notice patterns, start to summarise the common features, circumstances and triggers. Write these important factors down and have them handy as a reference point to help you identify what might be going on. You can use these as a guide in a vulnerable moment, or during the time you have set to reflect back on your journal.

These are some of the things Suki noticed:

- She tended to not eat a substantial breakfast, simply because she didn't make the time.
- On days when she tried to have a low-calorie lunch, and avoid carbohydrates, she was more likely to binge in the evening.
- Her children's dinners tended to be a particular trigger point, so on days when she was preparing these she needed to be aware of this.

- She was very hard on herself, often telling herself she'd failed or was greedy.
- "Sod it" was a common thought before binges.
- She felt guilty after eating food that she enjoyed.
- She often responded to the guilt of eating a "banned" food by engaging in a punishing exercise regime. Suki had to reflect on her exercise to really ask herself whether it was normal and healthy, or driven and excessive.

EXERCISE: WHAT ARE THE PATTERNS TO YOUR EATING PROBLEMS?

Consider if any of the below are playing a role in your day-to-day eating problem:

- Hunger
- Unpleasant emotions
- Energy levels
- Being disinhibited (alcohol or drug use?)
- Stressful situations
- Not making enough time
- Distressing body image thoughts
- Being alone

Anything else contributing to your eating problem:

COMMON PROBLEMS WITH JOURNALING

"I'll get worried/overwhelmed/upset by writing this down. It will make me feel worse."

Remember, this journal is not to be used to punish yourself. It may seem difficult to acknowledge your emotions or upsetting situations, but we have found that it's helpful to be honest with yourself. The more you become aware of your thoughts and feelings, the easier it will be. Sometimes, the simple act of writing these things down can take some of the heat out of the emotion, or help you to see things differently.

"I'll feel shame about what I've eaten."

If you are struggling to write down what you're eating, try to remind yourself that the aim is to be curious, not judgemental. Being faced with the facts can be painful initially, but in order to help overcome any eating problem, you need to know what you are eating and what's happening for you when you are using problematic eating behaviours. Be compassionate with yourself during this process. It is brave and you can be proud that you have even picked up this book and are willing to try to make change.

"I keep forgetting."

Try to make it part of your routine. At first you might need to use alarms or Post-It notes as a reminder. Alternatively, apps like Recovery Record have inbuilt reminders that you can set.

The process of facing and unpacking your eating behaviour can be really challenging. It takes courage to acknowledge there is a problem in the first place. However, this acknowledgement and detailed analysis of your eating is critical to being able to make changes and conquer your eating problems. Read on as we take you through a series of steps and tools that will help you along the journey.

CHAPTER 8

START REGULAR AND BALANCED EATING

Eating regularly is the cornerstone of overcoming eating problems. This is the case whether your main eating problem is under-eating or fear of eating, bingeing or out-of-control eating, or feeling like you have to compensate when you eat. There are so many physical and psychological benefits to eating regularly. While regular eating is not likely to be the whole answer to your eating problem, it is a vital first step.

> "When you are giving your body the fuel it needs, you are in a better position to tackle other elements of your eating problem."

When you are giving your body the fuel it needs during the day, you are in a better position to tackle any other elements of your eating problem that are relevant (such as emotional eating).

WHY EAT REGULARLY?

Have you ever noticed that trying to eat less during the day, or avoiding snacks and leaving big gaps without food, can sometimes lead to actually eating more? This isn't because you are "weak", but because your body desperately wants to eat regularly. Let's look at some reasons for this.

1. Regular eating reduces the likelihood of episodes of out-of-control eating.

Waiting longer than approximately four hours between a meal and snack can cause blood glucose levels to drop, hunger to increase, and result in extreme hunger and cravings. Unsurprisingly, if we skip a meal or snack, we tend to eat more at the next meal or snack. This can lead to eating more than usual, pushing past the sense of fullness, and even bingeing.

2. If you undereat and don't eat regularly enough, your metabolism may slow down and you might feel uncomfortably full when you do eat.

Eating regularly means your body begins to trust that you will feed it, and it will therefore process food more quickly. This means you won't feel as uncomfortable or bloated when you do eat (although some fullness after eating is normal).

3. Eating regularly feeds your mind.

Giving your body the nutrition it needs throughout the day helps you to think clearly and regulate your mood. This reduces the chances of you turning to food as a way of managing feelings.

4. Eating regularly will help you overcome anxiety you feel about eating.

Although it may sound counterintuitive, the only way to face your fears about eating is to eat regularly. This allows your body and mind to become comfortable with eating, and to see that catastrophic consequences do not occur.

5. Regular eating can make us feel more in control.

When we don't eat regularly, we become hungry and later feel more ravenous. This may lead you to eat past the point of comfortable fullness.

HOW TO EAT REGULARLY

Regular eating is eating every 2–4 hours, and incorporating 3 meals and 2–3 snacks each day.

Some key things to remember:

- Don't wait until you are hungry to eat. This may seem contrary to what you have been taught, but if you have been dieting, hunger and fullness signals can be all mixed up. You therefore can't rely on these signals to tell you when to eat. Your body is like a car; it needs to have fuel in the tank otherwise it will slow down and stop running. The emptier it is, the more fuel is needed to top it up.

- Plan ahead. Try to think of what you will eat for the day. You may want to make a plan in your journal so you can be sure you have the food you need available. You may also find making a weekly plan helpful.

- Make a shopping list, or do an online supermarket shop for the week. Try not to go to the supermarket every day, especially when you are hungry.

- If certain meals are trickier, e.g. your evening meal, try to plan these in advance. Batch-cook meals so you always have something readily available. Remember lots of foods can be frozen if you don't want to eat the same thing three days in a row, so use that freezer! If cooking is not your thing, or it feels too overwhelming, ready meals are another great option.

- If you tend to skip breakfast, get your breakfast ready the night before to save some time. This meal is so important.

- Plan around your social events. If you know you are going to be out and this will disrupt your eating plan, think about when and how you will ensure you have regular food around or during this event.

- Even if you are planning a big dinner out, stick with the regular eating plan during the day. Don't try to under-eat or compensate in anticipation of a big meal. One meal will not cause you to automatically gain weight, but restricting or compensating can lead to out-of-control eating later on.

- If you slip up with eating regularly, start the next meal afresh. Each new meal is a chance to get back on track.

HELPING YOURSELF WITH REGULAR EATING

Use loved ones for support. If regular eating feels like a giant leap, ask someone to sit and share a meal with you. It may also be wise to have someone support you afterwards if these are your most challenging times, due to unpleasant emotions (e.g. guilt, anxiety) or because you have urges to act in unhelpful ways (e.g. to vomit or excessively exercise). Like any new behaviour, it takes time to practise making change before it feels easier.

For example, Clare had skipped breakfast ever since she was in high school, so adding breakfast in was a massive challenge for her. But when she started having breakfast (as well as her morning snack) she noticed she was more energised and less obsessed with food during the day. She tackled breakfasts by initially having these later than most people would (i.e. 10.30am), but slowly bringing the time forward each day. She also found that having her cereal in a bowl ready the night before was a good visual reminder of what she needed to do.

There will be times when you are trying to eat regularly, but the pull of your eating problems is strong. Try to predict which moments you might find it difficult to stick with regular eating, and plan ways to stay on track at these times specifically. For example, you might notice that a bad day at work makes you feel stressed, or spending too much time on social media leads you to make more body comparisons than usual. In these situations, you may find regular eating really difficult, and you may be tempted to return to unhelpful eating behaviours (such as bingeing, extreme dieting). Try to prepare in advance for these situations.

Here are some ideas if you feel stuck with eating regularly:

- Note down which situations are likely to be difficult.
- Keep handy reminders of why it's important to eat regularly.
- If the problem is a loss of control over eating, try to postpone acting on this urge by 15 minutes and do something else. We have found that this is often enough to reduce the intensity of the urge itself. But of course if you haven't eaten enough in the day, no amount of distraction will help because your body is physiologically hungry.
- If you find it difficult to stop eating after you've had your planned meal or snack, then plan an activity for straight after you have eaten. Try to do something that means you leave the environment you were eating in, for example, going to another room. Also try to do something that occupies your mind, like a sudoku, talking to a friend or doing something you love. You might like to make a list of the activities that you could use to occupy your mind.
- If you find it difficult to continue with eating regularly because you are worried about your weight skyrocketing, then please see Chapter 17. If you are someone who weighs yourself frequently to manage your worry about weight gain, we strongly recommend not weighing yourself more than once per week. Doing so will only increase your anxiety about weight, and will not give you a meaningful representation of your weight pattern anyway.
- If you go off track then remind yourself that you've eaten regularly before (even if only briefly), and you can do it again. Each time you do this it will get a bit more familiar. Remember that each time you eat regularly, you are consolidating a new path forward. Even if there are blips, you are making progress!
- Draw on strengths you find helpful in different areas of life. When you've faced other challenges/blips, what do you do? How have you motivated and encouraged yourself to stay on track with exam preparation, for example?

Let's take a look at Suki and how she got on with regular eating. Suki had been really worrying that regular eating would make her gain weight, and so tried to skip meals. When people at work were talking about dieting, she found it particularly hard to stay on track with her meal plan and eat lunch. When Suki noticed that this was a pattern, she started to prepare her meals for the week in advance, and go out to the local park for her lunch break. She put a reminder on her phone to prompt her that it was lunchtime, and a note on her phone about why regular eating was so important to tackle her eating problems.

BALANCED EATING

Once you are eating *regularly*, you can start to tackle *what* you are eating to ensure you are incorporating all food groups. If eating particular foods/food groups has become very frightening for you, we cover this more extensively in Chapter 10. Below we offer some general guidance about balanced eating.

> "Once you are eating *regularly*, you can start to tackle *what* you are eating to ensure you are incorporating all food groups."

Some people aren't sure or can't remember a time when their eating was balanced, and have lost touch with what "normal" eating looks like. This means that you might not be able to tell if you have deprived yourself. If this is you, don't worry – this is something we commonly see.

To learn or re-learn an eating pattern that is sufficient and balanced, and to overcome deprivation, try these approaches:

- Ask yourself: when I *didn't* have eating problems, would I have eaten in this way?
- Look at what others who have a good relationship with food are eating. While everyone's exact dietary needs are not the same, it will give you a rough idea of whether you are depriving yourself.

- The information in Part I The Groundwork will give you the basis from which to work out what foods you need to be incorporating in a balanced diet, and why. Ask yourself whether you're including the full range of nutrition that your body needs.
- Have a look at our chapters on dieting and strict food rules. Experiment with making changes to your eating and see if this helps with reducing the problem eating. Some experiments might include: having a bigger breakfast, having a more sufficient snack, adding carbohydrates and fats to your meals, or adding foods that you enjoy to your day.
- If you have done these things and still need support and guidance about what a normal day's eating should look like for you, we encourage you to seek the support of a registered dietitian or nutritionist with expert knowledge in working with problem eating.

Regular and balanced eating is key to overcoming any eating problem. However, this often takes time to implement consistently. Keep heart! It is normal for there to be obstacles along the way. In the coming chapters we will explore some of these common obstacles.

CHAPTER 9

STOP COMPENSATORY BEHAVIOURS

Maybe your specific problem is related to using the
compensatory behaviours we have looked at earlier, such as
excessive exercise, vomiting, laxative or diet pill use, or fasting.
We have already covered how detrimental and ineffective these
behaviours are. Despite knowing this, they can be really difficult
to stop. Below we consider some skills that help interrupt and
hopefully eliminate these behaviours.

REGULAR EATING

When you respond to eating by using a compensatory behaviour,
you will soon become uncomfortable with the normal feelings
related to eating, such as fullness. When you eat regularly, the
feelings related to fullness are less extreme and you get used to
them. The first step is to practise tolerating these feelings, in
order for you to see that they pass with time.

If you are finding yourself consumed with your worries or on
your body as you are adjusting to regular eating, you may want to
use distracting activities. We would recommend that this is a short-
term tool at first, as relying on distraction when you eat could
become a form of unhelpful avoidance in the long term. More on
this later.

POSTPONE THE BEHAVIOUR

By postponing or delaying the compensatory behaviour, you are giving yourself some time to breathe and let the urge pass. Find something to do during this period when you have the urge to use these behaviours and see what happens. If the behaviour has become automatic, pausing can allow you to slow the cycle down and give you an opportunity to take another path. See if you can postpone even for a short time at first (such as five minutes) and gradually lengthen this out.

> "If the behaviour has become automatic, pausing can allow you to slow the cycle down and give you an opportunity to take another path."

GRADUALLY CUT DOWN THE FREQUENCY

If eliminating these behaviours feels really hard, make a start by working to reduce the frequency or amount of them. For example, if you feel you have an unhealthy standard of swimming a certain number of lengths, cut it down. Maybe you could trade exercise that feels punishing for more fun gym classes or something that is social. In any case, make a start by cutting down.

TELL YOUR SUPPORT CREW AND GET SUPPORT

We get that these behaviours might be so deeply personal for you – and might even feel embarrassing to share. But, as we have mentioned, getting support from others is helpful both emotionally (if you are having a bad day) and practically (if you want company for moments when you are more likely to engage in these behaviours).

FIND SOMETHING ELSE TO DO

Fill your time and mind with other things that can distract you. Call a friend, take a walk, do a crossword – anything to help you shift focus.

PREPARE FOR WHAT YOU MIGHT STRUGGLE WITH

You might have been using these behaviours for so long that you feel you are on autopilot. However, you might also be using them to manage difficult thoughts or feelings. If so, when you don't use the behaviours, you will find in the short term that you will have to face these thoughts and feelings instead. This is uncomfortable but is actually progress! Have a look at Chapters 12 to 16 for some ideas of how to deal with this, if it does happen.

BIN THE LAXATIVES/DIET PILLS

If you have made the choice that you don't want to take these behaviours into the future, bin the laxatives or diet pills now. There is no time like the present.

A word of caution: if you suddenly stop taking laxatives, water retention can occur as fluid levels return to normal, and this can cause bloating or swelling of the feet and ankles (which can last up to 10–14 days after stopping). Get support from your doctor to gradually reduce the number and frequency of laxatives used to avoid this.

Changing these behaviours is difficult and rarely happens overnight. Give each of these strategies a go to see which work best for you as you continue with other aspects of overcoming your eating problem. In the next chapter, we will be looking at a key maintaining feature of most eating problems, and one that is critical to address in order to help you move forward: strict eating rules.

CHAPTER 10

ABANDON STRICT FOOD RULES

By now you might have realised that to overcome your eating problem, it is not your body that needs to change, but your mind.

People with eating problems often talk about trying to stick to "food rules". These rules are different to guidelines as they tend to be black and white, feel impossible to wiggle out of, and if broken are usually followed by feelings of guilt, frustration and disappointment. They can be rules about particular foods, food groups, or eating-related situations (such as the timing of eating). Overly strict food rules drive a lot of problem eating. They masquerade as the answer to the eating problem, but most of the time they only make the problem worse.

Food rules can come from a variety of sources. Perhaps you picked one up from the media, or from a friend – something like "I must avoid all refined sugar." Or you read an article that promised a fantasy of painless weight loss and immediate happiness – and encouraged you to avoid all carbohydrates. Maybe it's a rule that relates to your own experience and serves to protect you from certain emotions, like "If I eat cake, I will feel guilty, so I must avoid it."

> "Overly strict food rules drive a lot of problem eating. They masquerade as the answer to the eating problem, but most of the time they only make the problem worse."

Some people also observe certain fasting practices, avoid certain foods or animal products for cultural, ethical or religious reasons, or have a medically prescribed diet. Of course, this is not a problem so long as the *motivation* is healthy. Thinking about motivation is key.

DO YOU HAVE STRICT FOOD RULES?

Typically, strict food rules are unhelpful. However, it's normal and healthy to have guidelines about eating that you flexibly adhere to, with the aim of overall health in mind.

So, how do you know if your rule is a help or a hindrance? It might help to ask yourself the following questions:

- Are you more rigid with your food rules than those around you?
- Do you think of any food as "bad", "forbidden", or "dangerous"? Or do you think of others as "good" or "clean"?
- How would you feel if you had to break one of your food rules? For example, if you eat the same cereal every morning, could you eat something else if you were a guest at someone's house? Or could you eat a variety of things from a breakfast buffet?
- Do you feel you *must* compensate if you don't adhere to a rule?
- Are you using the word "should" or "must" rather than "would like to" about a food or eating behaviour?
- How much does it impact your life to try to stick to your rules? Do you have to make sacrifices or go out of your way?
- What thoughts does breaking the rule bring up for you? Are they critical thoughts about yourself?

BANNED FOODS

You may have found that over time you have completely avoided certain foods due to fear of what will happen if you eat them. A lot of people have developed a subconscious or conscious list of "good" and "bad" foods. "Bad" foods tend to be thought of as "junk" foods. This is a really unhelpful term as actually all foods can be enjoyed and incorporated into a nutritionally balanced diet. Even these foods have nutritional value, whether

"'Bad' foods tend to be thought of as 'junk' foods. This is a really unhelpful term as actually all foods can be enjoyed and incorporated into a nutritionally balanced diet."

it be energy from carbohydrate and sugar, or various vitamins and minerals that are contained within their components, e.g. calcium from foods containing dairy. In overcoming strict food rules, one of the scariest things might be learning to eat these foods again, but this is vital to improving our relationship with food. It is only when we realise that *all* foods have value that we can start listening to what our body wants and needs and start eating without guilt and anxiety.

EAT CLEAN OR EAT DIRTY?

"Clean eating" deserves a mention here. In recent years, this term has become synonymous with health and wellness, and has become a popular if not an acceptable way to eat. The problem is: when was eating ever dirty? These words themselves are laden with right vs wrong, good vs bad and virtue vs guilt (otherwise known as "black and white thinking"). We have seen an increase in those adopting clean eating practices in recent years under the guise of health, wellness and nutrition. However, clean eaters can be far from healthy and, from both a physical and psychological perspective, may be in a cycle of deprivation and food and body obsession.

If you adopt a clean eating pattern, ask yourself: would you follow clean eating practices if they made you gain weight? If your

> "If you adopt a clean eating pattern, ask yourself: would you follow clean eating practices if they made you gain weight? If your answer is no, then perhaps have a think about the motivation behind this way of eating."

answer is no, then perhaps have a think about the motivation behind this way of eating.

A new term that has been coined because of this rise in healthy eating obsession is "Orthorexia". Although not yet a clinical diagnosis, it is commonly seen in people with problem eating. The National Eating Disorders Association have noted the following warning signs[5]:

- Compulsive checking of nutritional labels
- Increased concern about the health of ingredients
- Cutting out an increasing number of food groups (i.e. all sugar, all carbs, all dairy, all meat, all animal products)
- Inability to eat anything but a narrow group of foods that are deemed "healthy" or "pure"
- Unusual interest in the health of what others are eating
- Spending hours per day thinking about what food might be served at upcoming events
- Showing high levels of distress when "safe" or "healthy" foods aren't available
- Obsessive following of food and "healthy lifestyle" blogs on social media

The obsession around healthy eating is framed as a lifestyle choice but is essentially another diet governed by food rules. It takes us away from listening to what our body wants and needs and adopts a virtuous stance to food choices, taking the "you

[5] National Eating Disorders Association (2018). *Orthorexia*. Available at: www.nationaleatingdisorders.org/learn/by-eating-disorder/other/orthorexia [Accessed 30 July 2020].

are what you eat" phrase literally! When the rules are broken, it does not just result in feelings of guilt and shame, but also feels as though it is a reflection on the kind of person you are. Some social media accounts can really buy into this approach to food without robust evidence.

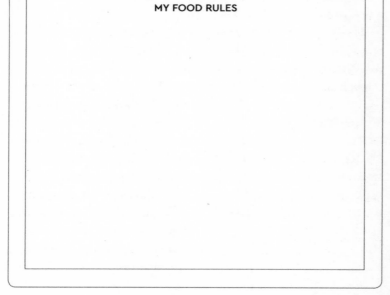

EXERCISE: YOUR FOOD RULES

Take some time now to list your food rules and think about your reason for each one. Is the rule motivated by shape and weight? Do you have a strong emotional response if you think about letting go of this rule? Once you have done this, rank them in order of how strongly each are held.

For example, one of Suki's rules is "I must not eat carbohydrates". Among Clare's are "I must eat less than 1,500 calories per day," and "I shouldn't eat past 6pm". Chris attempts to follow the rule "I must not eat in front of my colleagues, or I will be considered greedy".

MY FOOD RULES

CALORIE-COUNTING RULES

For a long time, society has focused on a mathematical equation:

energy in - energy out = weight maintenance

According to this equation, as long as we match our exercise to the amount we eat, or ensure that we are in calorie deficit, we can control our weight.

The idea of calorie control has permeated society, to the point that all packaged food has nutritional information easily visible. Many restaurants also have the calories plastered on the menu. It is no wonder that this has led to our calorie obsession. More and more people are counting and comparing calories, using calorie and activity trackers, and recording food and exercise on phone apps to try to ensure on a daily basis that calorie balance or deficit is being achieved.

In broad terms, yes, if we consistently eat much more than we expend over an extended period of time, we will have a surplus of energy, which will cause weight gain. But it is not as black and white as this and, not surprisingly, our bodies are not as simple as a mathematical equation.

The "energy in" bit is the food we eat, but the "energy out" part is not just the exercise we do, but all of the processes in the body that use energy. We cannot accurately calculate these bodily processes through an equation or phone app, and these processes are different every day. Some days we will be using more energy and other days less. Our bodies are really great at responding to this by increasing or decreasing our hunger signals. Also, on days we are eating less, our metabolism can slow down, which means despite eating less and being in "negative energy balance", it will

"The more we adhere to external food rules, the more we disconnect from our body's internal cues, and the harder it is and the longer it takes to get these back."

not result in weight loss. This also occurs on days where we might eat more. For example, at a party or a nice meal, our body can adapt to being in "positive energy balance" by speeding up our metabolism, *which is why one meal or one day will not cause big changes in our weight.*

The biggest danger with calorie counting is that it is just another set of rules to help us decide what and how much to eat. The more we adhere to external food rules, the more we disconnect from our body's internal cues, and the harder it is and the longer it takes to get these back.

OVERCOMING STRICT FOOD RULES

When we are anxious about something, we tend to avoid it. The more you avoid the things you're afraid of, the more afraid of them you become.

If you are afraid of what will happen when you eat a certain food or are in certain situations, then it's understandable that you will want to avoid those foods or settings. You might create rules about foods to manage your anxiety. But if you have banned foods or "no go" eating-related situations, then eating might have an unhealthy control in your life.

"If you have banned foods or 'no go' eating-related situations, then eating might have an unhealthy control in your life."

If this is you, try to slowly face your fears by gradually introducing some of these avoided or banned foods into your diet. This is a difficult task, and we appreciate it might feel scary or even unnecessary. However, we think it can be really helpful in order to loosen the anxiety around eating, food, shape and weight.

EXERCISE: ANXIETY-PROVOKING FOODS

To gradually face fears, you need to map out what a path forward would look like. That means figuring out what makes you a bit anxious (you avoid it sometimes), and what makes you super anxious (you avoid it completely).

To help with this, create a hierachy of foods ranging from those you eat with no anxiety to those that make you very anxious and you currently avoid. If there are whole food groups in here, break them up further. For example, if carbohydrates on the whole make you feel anxious, think about whether there is any difference in anxiety level for specific carbohydrates (e.g. what about rice, pasta, bread, potatoes?). Then add in eating-related situations that also make you anxious. Are there particular times of day you feel more nervous to eat? Or particular social situations?

See Clare's example below of her anxiety-provoking foods:

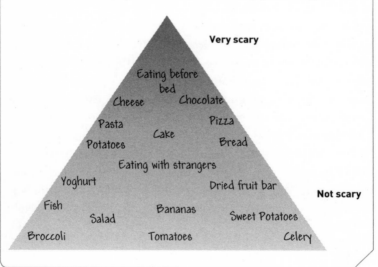

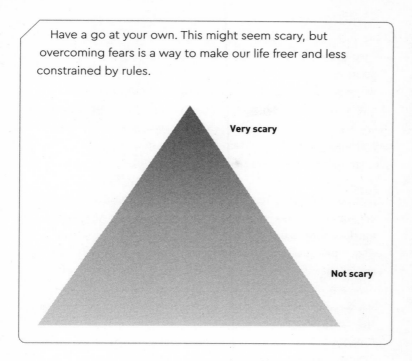

Have a go at your own. This might seem scary, but overcoming fears is a way to make our life freer and less constrained by rules.

Very scary

Not scary

Try to see gradually including these foods and situations as a positive challenge that moves you towards the life you want to live – free of eating problems. Give it a go... what is there to lose?

EVALUATING DIETARY GUIDANCE

Because there is such an array of information immediately available to us these days, we understand why many people find themselves consulting websites and social media to find answers about health and wellbeing. The internet is a great resource, but equally can be a confusing vortex of information! "Doctor Google" also has no quality control. Despite us not knowing anything about quantum physics, any one of us could write an article about it and upload it to the Internet. Similarly, many well-intended bloggers and social media influencers may write about food and eating, with the content varying hugely in quality and expertise.

Some of you may have found yourself in this situation and could even now be feeling more confused about food and eating. Maybe you thought diets were the answer, or that you should eat clean. Maybe you read somewhere that certain food groups are bad. If you're feeling confused about how to know what's true, here are some tips to find reliable information:

- Does the person giving advice have any commercial interest? An example of this would be somebody selling a weight-loss product, who is also sponsored by that product.
- Check the qualifications of the person who is giving you the advice. Are they a qualified health professional, registered with their professional body? Are they a generalist, or are they a specialist in that field? Is the advice they're giving within their specialist area and expertise?
- Are they claiming scientific evidence of a viewpoint by sharing *only* anecdotal (personal experience) evidence? Or are they reporting the findings of robust, controlled, scientific studies? (For more information on the importance of rigorous science, read *Bad Science* by Ben Goldacre (2009)).
- Remember, if it seems too good to be true, it probably is...

We hope that you have been able to reflect on the rules that you might possess that could be maintaining your eating problem. Understandably, you might be reluctant to give these up. If so, we hope that the next section, which tackles our thoughts and behaviours related to food might give you more specific and practical tools and strategies to help equip you to move forward.

PART III

GET EQUIPPED

CHAPTER 11

IT'S ALL ABOUT PERCEPTION

We all see the world differently and interpret the same situation in our own unique way. Our personality, our upbringing and our experiences all affect the way we see things. This includes how we see food and how we see our bodies.

Often, we hear people talk about how they are feeling day to day and how a situation made them feel. For example, Suki might arrive at home and say to her partner, "I've had a dreadful day because I went to a lunch meeting and all they served was pasta." However, there is another aspect of Suki's experience which is the part we want you to examine more clearly – her thoughts.

In Suki's case, she arrived at the meeting, saw the pasta meal and *thought*, "I can't eat pasta. I'm going to blow my diet. I'm going to gain so much weight if I eat it." Suki's thoughts had contributed to her overall experience of feeling worry and unhappiness about the lunch meeting. However in the initial stages of her treatment, she was hardly aware of this mental chatter that was happening in her mind all day long, affecting her emotions and her behaviour.

> "Our personality, our upbringing and our experiences all affect the way we see things. This includes how we see food and how we see our bodies."

As we don't all see things in the same way, we want to spend some time now exploring how your perceptions and thoughts can be influencing your own eating problems.

SO, HOW CAN WE UNDERSTAND OUR THOUGHTS?

Thoughts can be positive, negative or neutral; unhelpful or helpful; accurate or inaccurate; fast or slow. We all perceive situations to be something that they are not sometimes. This happens partly because we are all unique human beings with our own stories and experiences that colour how we interpret our day-to-day experiences. It also happens because we are all constantly trying to process information, and our brain does this so quickly that sometimes it makes mistakes.

"Remember: Just because you think it, doesn't make it true."

Take, for example, this thought: "I'm hungry. I haven't eaten since lunch." This has likely been triggered by what you are seeing/hearing/experiencing in the present moment and is factual. Compare this to the thoughts "I'm hungry because I'm greedy" or "It's obvious to everyone I've gained weight this week" arise from a combination of situational factors and what you are experiencing inside. These latter thoughts are skewed as a result of background fears, insecurities, or a tendency to misinterpret certain experiences.

We will explore some of the particular thinking biases we can have later, but for now it's important to know that we can certainly have untrue and unhelpful thoughts.

Remember: Just because you think it, doesn't make it true.

Being fully aware that not all your thoughts are true is the first step to thinking differently. A common metaphor is to think of our minds as being like the sky and our thoughts like clouds – they are always coming and going, changing shape, intensity and frequency. The sky encompasses the clouds, but is not solely composed of them. In the same way, our minds do not need to be ruled by our thoughts, even when they feel strong and tumultuous. Instead, you can become a curious observer of your mind. Read on to see how.

COGNITIVE BEHAVIOURAL THERAPY

We all have untrue and unhelpful thoughts sometimes and they can have a real impact on us. When these thoughts become especially intense or really frequent, they can interfere in our lives – leading us to do things we want to stop or change.

Cognitive behavioural therapy, or CBT, is a type of therapy that looks at how your thoughts are associated with your emotions, your behaviours, and your physiological sensations (feelings in your body). It focuses on how we think about and interpret our experiences, and helps us adapt these thoughts and change the associated problem behaviours and emotional experiences.

The first step in CBT is to become more aware of your own thinking. We are hopeful that through completing the journal we recommended in Chapter 7, you might have already begun to notice some of your interpretations and thinking patterns.

AUTOMATIC THOUGHTS

Like Suki, it's often easier to be aware of how a situation makes us feel, but not as easy to figure out what we are thinking. This is because our initial thoughts happen quickly, and are well rehearsed, which makes us pretty used to them. In CBT, we call these initial thoughts our "automatic thoughts" because of how immediate, subconscious and unstoppable they are. When we tune into and catch our thoughts, we begin to realise the impact they have on how we feel and what we do.

Left unquestioned, we act as if our automatic thoughts are true. If the thoughts and feelings were negative, then we might be more inclined to act in an unhelpful way in order to make ourselves feel better. These actions then have consequences of their own, and often make the whole cycle of negative automatic thoughts

"The more you act as if these automatic thoughts are true, the more true they feel."

recur again and again. The more you act as if these automatic thoughts are true, the more true they feel.

Take the example of a colleague (who you have a good relationship with) walking straight past you in the corridor at work without acknowledging you. There are a variety of different ways one could interpret this situation. An automatic thought of "They didn't acknowledge me because they don't like me" or "They think I'm useless at my job" will lead to an emotional response of anxiety or sadness, and perhaps a behaviour of avoiding that person to prevent that feeling of anxiety or sadness again. By avoiding your colleague, it is likely that you will have more frequent thoughts about your colleague not liking you. This is because avoiding them means you're not getting any information to the contrary. Now, of course, there is always the possibility that the colleague might not like you. But, from this behaviour in the corridor alone, you cannot be sure. Conversely, you might have the thought "They seemed preoccupied, I hope they are okay", in which case you are more likely to have a feeling of concern for them, and the urge to ask them how they are. By checking in with them, you have a chance to get a more realistic interpretation of why they didn't acknowledge you.

Put simply, it isn't the colleague walking past you that inherently creates the bad feeling, it's *how you interpret* that situation. How we think dictates how we feel and what we do. Interpreting ambiguous events negatively leads to unpleasant feelings and often to negative cycles of unhelpful behaviour as we respond to our interpretation.

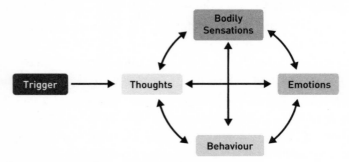

Adapted from Greenberger and Padesky, 1995[6]

---

[6]   Greenberger, D. & Padesky, C. A. (1995). *Mind over mood: A cognitive therapy treatment manual for clients.* Guilford Press: New York, NY, US.

Let's look at an eating-related example:

Clare follows a fairly restrictive diet, and when her friend made her a cake for her birthday, she had the automatic thought "I shouldn't have that, I will get fat." In Clare's case, this thought led to unpleasant emotions, including anxiety and disgust, as well as unpleasant feelings in her body as her heart raced and she felt a drop in her stomach. When she had these emotions and bodily sensations, Clare tried to manage them by avoiding the birthday cake.

Unfortunately, avoiding the cake reinforces this cycle, making it more likely that Clare will feel anxious about cake in the future and, therefore, continue to avoid it. For Clare, the thought of cake leads to her feeling anxious, but for someone else, being offered a slice of cake could lead to another emotion, such as excitement, curiosity or maybe disappointment (if the flavour was not their preference). The difference will depend on what we *think* about birthday cake in the first place.

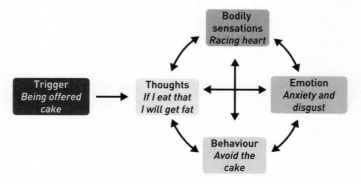

Clare's friends have started to notice her eating patterns. She is becoming more and more upset by the way she thinks about eating, and the way she deprives herself of food that she enjoys. This pattern is also having an impact on her relationships with people, who believe that it is entirely acceptable (indeed, enjoyable) to have cake to celebrate a birthday. Not to mention they are feeling a bit miffed that she didn't even try a slice, given that they had prepared it especially for her. As well as allowing herself the cake, Clare knew that she needed to manage her thoughts differently to feel better. She needed to first "catch" these unhelpful thoughts.

For a moment, think about the negative thoughts that are particularly troublesome for you. The ones that your mind fixates on and that lead to emotions that are unpleasant. These thoughts could be related to the way you see the world, yourself or other people.

EXERCISE: NOTICING NEGATIVE THOUGHTS

Some people find it difficult to identify their thoughts. If this is you, a useful way to catch these thoughts is to complete a diary. You might have already noticed some of your thoughts and how they relate to your emotions in the moment, from keeping your journal. However, this task requires you to dig deeper into the specific thoughts you have that drive your emotions and behaviours.

What's the situation?

What were your thoughts?

How did you feel?

What did you feel in your body?

What did you do?

As you can see, the way you think about things is closely linked to how you feel and how you act. These factors might explain why you are in a cycle of problematic eating that has felt difficult to break. In the following chapters we explore these thoughts even more, looking at how you can break the cycle by tackling your thoughts, feelings and behaviours. We start with tackling unhelpful thoughts.

CHAPTER 12

ADDRESSING HOW WE THINK

Remember that mantra from the last chapter: Just because you think it, doesn't make it true. Thoughts are not facts. By uncovering what your negative automatic thoughts are and looking at what problems might be occurring in how you are thinking, you can target and manage the unhelpful and untrue thoughts. The goal here is not *positive* thinking, but *realistic* thinking. By focusing on realistic thinking, we believe you will be less likely to experience unpleasant emotions, and hopefully act in a way that is helpful to you.

> "The goal here is not *positive* thinking, but *realistic* thinking."

It can be hard to figure out whether our thoughts are true or not, especially if we have thought a certain way for a long time. We might have come to believe something is true, even if it's not.

Below are some ideas of how you can respond when you notice those negative thoughts. Use these to give yourself a chance to see things in a new way.

QUESTION YOUR THINKING

In order to check out the accuracy of how you think about a situation, you need to be curious and open-minded while looking at your thoughts. Some helpful questions to ask yourself when you evaluate your thinking include:

- Is there any other way I could view this situation?
- Are there any other possible explanations?

- Is there anything I am ignoring about the situation?
- Would I say this to a friend? If this happened to a friend, would I interpret it in the same way?
- If I was sitting a test in which I was scored on how accurate my thoughts were, would I submit this thought as an answer?
- What would I tell a younger person confronted with the same scenario? What would I say to a child?

THINKING STYLES

Once you have tuned into the way you think, or interpret events, you can start to consider the various patterns to your thinking. These patterns can contribute to us misinterpreting events, or seeing events in a way that causes distress. It's therefore important to notice when you do this. Below is a list of some common problematic thinking styles as they relate to eating behaviours. Have a read and identify the ones that are most relevant for you.

- **Catastrophising.** Thinking the worst-case scenario in situations. Example: *"If I eat out with my friend, I won't be able to control myself and will eat the whole buffet"* or *"What if after my appraisal I lose my job?"*
- **Crystal Ball Gazing.** Predicting the future with your thoughts even without this outcome happening before. Example: *"Everyone will think I'm greedy if I order a pizza"* or *"I am going to put on so much weight after that burger."*
- **Black-and-White Thinking.** Thinking in all-or-nothing terms, with no shades of grey. Example: *"Carbohydrates are bad"* or *"If my weight isn't under 9 stone, I have failed."*
- **Jumping to Conclusions.** Making an immediate judgement about a situation without proof. Example: *"These jeans didn't fit me, so all jeans will look bad on me"* or *"They haven't returned my call because they don't care about me."*

- **Should-ing and Must-ing.** Telling yourself that you "should" or "must" do things, as opposed to "could" or "might".
  Example: *"I shouldn't eat anything sweet for the whole of January as this will make me gain weight" or "I shouldn't feel upset."*
- **Mind Reading.** Assuming that you know what someone else is thinking.
  Example: *"All my colleagues think I am fat and lazy" or "My boss wants to fire me."*
- **Labelling.** Using a derogatory label for yourself or others. Speaking in global terms about yourself or others, not considering variability in who you/others are.
  Example: *"I am ugly and useless" or "I'm weak because I didn't stick to the diet."*
- **Emotional Reasoning.** Thinking that the way you feel must make your perception of something true.
  Example: *"I feel so overweight, so I must be" or "I feel like they're angry with me, so they must be."*
- **Minimising.** Under-stating or dismissing the importance of something.
  Example: *"I managed regular eating on two out of seven days, which isn't enough" or "They are only telling me I looked nice at the gala ball because they feel sorry for me."*
- **Personalising.** Taking things personally and thinking that you are the reason, or responsible, for most things. Not considering other causes that contribute to a situation.
  Example: *"They didn't serve pudding at the dinner party because they think I don't need it" or "The comment about the team needing to increase productivity at work was about me."*
- **Tunnel Vision.** Zooming in on one part of a situation rather than considering the whole situation. Usually this means picking up negative parts and not noticing the positive.
  Example: *"Everyone at the party was noticing what I ate"* (based on just one comment from one person who said they also liked the cake they saw me eating).

Once you've read these, put a mark beside your top three – the ones you do the most. Remember, all of our minds naturally fall into these thinking styles at times! Our brains are trying throughout the day to process so much information as quickly as possible, and so sometimes biases slip in. Our goal is just to notice what biases our mind tends to lean towards.

Once you have identified your top three, notice when your mind comes up with thoughts that match these thinking styles. Write these on a card you carry around with you, put the list on a note on your phone, or pin it to a pinboard in your room. Every day, ask yourself: to what extent have I been engaging in [insert your thinking style] today?

TAKE THE THOUGHT TO COURT

Imagine that the thought causing you distress is on trial in a court of law. There is a lawyer defending the thought, in this case bringing all the evidence that the thought is true. There is another lawyer prosecuting the thought, bringing all the evidence that this thought is not true. Remember, in a court of law, only facts that are accepted as true can be submitted as evidence. Having a "feeling" about something is not evidence enough. Imagine what a judge would say to that!

Take Clare's thought, "I'll get fat if I eat the birthday cake", for example. She imagined this thought was in a court of law and wrote down the evidence for and against this thought:

Evidence for:
- Cake has calories so can result in weight gain
- Cake has sugar and fats in it

Evidence against:
- Eating one piece of cake does not result in automatic weight gain
- My body will use the calories to help me think and function

- I know I tend to worry about things that aren't based in reality; this could be why I'm having this thought
- Others around me eat cake in moderation and don't seem to gain weight
- I've eaten cake before and my weight didn't drastically change; I am "jumping to conclusions" again

Clare then looked over the evidence for and against this thought and weighed up the quality of her evidence. Having done this, she came up with a conclusion: that the cake would result in her taking in calories but a slice of cake would not result in permanent weight gain.

EXERCISE: TEST THE EVIDENCE

Now it's your turn. Write down the thought that is causing you distress or problems below:

Now consider the evidence for and against:

Evidence For	Evidence Against

Having weighed up the evidence for and against, what do you now think of how true your thought is?

Is there an alternative more accurate thought? What is it?

CONTINUUM THINKING

One of the most common problems about how we think is when we make black-and-white statements. This is particularly common in eating problems, where people repeatedly condemn themselves harshly and unfairly with labels like "greedy", "lazy", "stupid" and "ugly".

These are extreme statements, and we bet you would never say them to a friend. One way to overcome the extreme is by looking at the full range of what a word really means. For example, if "greediness" was on a continuum from 0 to 100, with 0 being not at all greedy and 100 being completely greedy, then what would it *really* mean if you are saying "I am greedy"? What does a person who is 100% greedy look like? Can you think of an example of the greediest person on the planet? Perhaps, to help give perspective, think about how you would teach the concept of greediness to a younger person.

Now, where does your "greed" level really fit in relation to this? The situation that led you to proclaim "I'm greedy" – is it up there with the 100%? Or are you unfairly labelling yourself? Is there a more moderate way of interpreting the situation that led you to make this absolute statement?

TALK TO YOUR SUPPORT CREW

Early on in this book, we talked about the importance of your support crew. When you find yourself caught in a negative thinking cycle, your friends, family and supporters really matter. Check out your worries with others. If they are nurturing and supportive people, who have your best interests at heart, their advice should be trustworthy. Also, an ability on their part to be objective will help if you are feeling confused and unsure. Talking out your thoughts can also help more with problem-solving, if needed.

The people you choose to talk to are paramount. Be aware if your conversations become circular and actually reinforce the thought, however. You really want your friend to be firm (in a warm way) to highlight to you when your thoughts are inaccurate or biased. Ask yourself whether the person you share your thinking with will be helpful and whether they will give you some rational perspective.

CATCH THE DIFFERENT INFORMATION

Frustratingly, it's very easy for us to notice the things that confirm (or *feel* as though they confirm) our negative thoughts. It's much harder for us to notice the evidence for the alternative, more balanced and helpful thoughts! This is called selective attention, and it's a normal process when we've thought a certain way for a long time. For the sake of ease, our brain tries to make new situations fit into the pattern that it knows. Even if that pattern is wrong! This means it's harder work to correct any errors in our thinking. We have to make a conscious effort to get a more comprehensive and realistic view of the situation, and that requires us to pay particular attention to evidence that goes *against* our negative automatic thought.

EXERCISE: EXPLORE ALTERNATIVE THOUGHTS

To help with developing and practising new, more balanced ways of seeing things, it can be helpful to keep a log or jot down times when you notice evidence that your negative automatic thought *isn't* true. Or evidence that a more balanced alternative thought *is* true. In other words, selectively attend to that evidence – not just the evidence that might support a negative thought.

Thought that causes me distress:

Evidence I have been relying on to "prove" this thought:

Is this evidence of good quality?

Can the evidence be seen in another way?

Are there any thinking biases inherent in this evidence?

What evidence to the contrary might I have been dismissing?

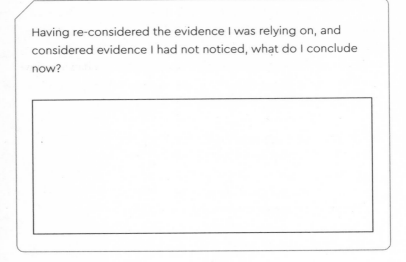

Having re-considered the evidence I was relying on, and considered evidence I had not noticed, what do I conclude now?

For example, Chris had a pattern of catastrophising, and these catastrophic thoughts fuelled his eating problem. During his job as a teacher, he was often given direct feedback from his boss about what he needed to do differently. He began to think, "They think I'm useless, they're going to fire me" when he got that feedback. These difficult thoughts and feelings fuelled urges to comfort eat to distract himself when he got home.

As time went on, he found himself dwelling on the critical feedback, feeling "useless" and becoming more and more convinced he would be fired. This was paralysing for Chris. The more tired he felt, the more these pieces of feedback felt like certain evidence that he would soon be fired.

After a discussion with his partner, however, Chris started to wonder whether he was *definitely* interpreting this work situation accurately. He already had a long list of examples that he felt backed up his belief that he would be fired. It turned out, however, that he'd been ignoring a lot of evidence to the contrary. When he began to purposefully notice, he found out that his colleagues all got the same amount of feedback. He also had a conversation with a colleague and discovered that the feedback style of his boss was blunt, and this wasn't personal to him. Chris also began to notice positive feedback that he had previously overlooked. When Chris took on board this contrary evidence that he was secure in his job, he began to feel more settled and less anxious when he got home. This in turn had a positive impact on his eating, with less urge to comfort eat when he got home.

Here's how Chris answered the questions in the Explore Alternative Thoughts exercise:

Thought that causes me distress:
They think I'm useless, they're going to fire me.

Evidence:
I have been relying on to "prove" this thought: Direct feedback at work about things I need to do differently.

Is this evidence of good quality?
It *feels* really true, but on a logical level I know that it's not really. Feedback does not equal firing. The interpretation I've made is just one possible interpretation.

Can it be seen in another way?
It's possible I'm getting feedback because they value me as an employee and want to help me develop my teaching style.

Are there any thinking biases inherent in this "evidence"?
Catastrophising, crystal ball gazing, personalising, mind reading.

What evidence to the contrary might I have been dismissing?
My colleagues all get a lot of feedback too. The person giving feedback has a reputation for giving blunt feedback, which is more about them than me. I also get positive feedback about my teaching.

Having considered this for a week, what do I conclude now?
I currently have no firm evidence I am going to be fired. Everyone gets feedback in my workplace. I do some things well and there are some things I can improve on. It is part of my boss' role to give me this type of feedback. On the whole, I'm doing a good job and there is no reason for me to worry about being fired.

INVEST IN THOUGHTS THAT ARE TRUE AND HELPFUL

In the same way that investing in negative and unhelpful thoughts will fuel negative and unhelpful behaviours in your life, if you invest in thoughts that are true and helpful, you will be more likely to act in a constructive way. For example, once you have decided to eat regularly and allow yourself previously forbidden foods, then nurture that thought. Invest in this new way of thinking by allowing yourself to eat all foods, knowing that this will help you to have a healthy relationship with food. Not to mention, it will help you live a life you feel satisfied with! You will find that the thoughts you invest in and nurture become more frequent, and the thoughts you dismiss as untrue or unhelpful become less common.

PRACTISE, PRACTISE, PRACTISE

Adopting new, realistic ways of thinking takes time. While you are in the process of practising your new evidence-based alternative thoughts and they're not coming to you naturally, try to make these easily accessible for yourself externally. Use cue cards, write on your mirror, put reminders on your phone or use Post-It notes. Do anything that will remind you of these thoughts to help you on your journey.

Through this chapter, we hope you have been able to examine your own patterns of thinking and notice when your thoughts are not true or helpful. Left unchallenged these thoughts can really drive unhelpful behavioural and emotional patterns, which are at the heart of a poor relationship with food. We have looked at how you can challenge thoughts that have been causing you difficulty, and develop evidence-based alternatives. Next, we will look at more general underlying rules, assumptions and beliefs that drive our thinking and can keep us stuck.

CHAPTER 13

RULES AND BELIEFS

We have been talking about how we interpret day-to-day situations. Often, though, there are other thoughts or fears that drive these habitual ways of thinking. Take, for example, the thought "If I don't monitor my weight, it will skyrocket." Underlying this thought could be the belief that "If I gain weight, I'll be unattractive," which could also be associated with an underlying fear that "I'll be alone."

There are different levels to our thinking, and we want to explore these a bit more. So first, let's take a look at what *drives* our automatic thoughts, and why we are inclined to think in our particular way.

WHAT ARE YOUR RULES FOR LIFE?

We avoid our underlying fears in life by developing rules for ourselves about how to live. These rules tend to be black and white, and not following them can lead to feeling worried, guilty or a sense of failure. Think of rules as our *self-imposed prerequisites* to living and the things we want to achieve. As already discussed, for someone with eating problems, rules are often related to eating habits as well as shape and weight. Some example rules are: "If I eat what I want, others won't like me" or "If I want to be happy, I cannot gain weight" or "To be in control of my life, I must be in control of my eating." Notice how black and white these rules sound!

But, rules related to eating and weight are often linked to more general rules. For example, a rule of being in control of your eating might be linked more broadly to rules such as the following: you must always be in control, meet others' expectations, put others first, and never let emotions get the better of you. It is worthwhile to explore whether the rules you have are helpful in overcoming your eating problem, or if these rules need to be left behind.

Check out some rules we commonly hear below and see if any are relevant to you. These rules are likely to be in addition to some strict food rules we looked at in Chapter 10. Remember, there is an infinite number of possible rules, so add any you have to the list.

- I must keep my weight below a certain number to be attractive
- I need to say yes to not upset others
- I must always eat less than others around me to feel in control
- I must be the thinnest of my friends to be respected
- I mustn't let my emotions get out of control or I'll go mad
- I must never show emotions to others or I'll be rejected
- I'll only be attractive if I'm thin
- I'll only be loved if I'm thin
- I must be in control at all times
- I won't cope with being out of control
- I need to weigh myself daily to check I haven't gained weight
- I must

  _____

- I must not

  _____

- I need to

  _____

Clare's eating problem was fuelled by an underlying rule that "In order to be successful, I need to control and restrict my eating." This would mean that during her day-to-day life, when faced with sugary foods, she would avoid these, as she assumed that this had a direct impact on her sense of success. Of course, objectively, we know this is not the case and that things that might be more commonly associated with success include working hard, meaningful relationships and having a good work/life balance. However, for Clare, these rules felt strong, fixed and vital for a sense of success and achievement.

WHAT TO DO ABOUT THESE RULES

If you've realised you're living by some black-and-white rules, we recommend you have a think about how you could adapt them so that you continue to free yourself from your eating problems.

So, how do you adapt these rules? Well, pretty much the same way you have done with your thinking in the previous chapter. Ask yourself, would this be a rule I would impose on others? Is this a fact or a feeling? Does this rule have any basis in reality? What are the pros and cons of this rule?

For Clare, becoming aware that the problem wasn't how much she was eating, but her misguided *rule*, was key. She was then able to focus on reaching for feelings of success in other ways. This led her to become more open to changing her relationship with food, as she realised that her success was truly dependent on other factors. She also tested this rule out by eating more in a regular and balanced way. As you might expect, she noticed that her success did not decrease by eating more. On the contrary, her achievement in so many areas of her life increased as she properly fuelled her body and mind.

"For Clare, becoming aware that the problem wasn't how much she was eating, but her misguided *rule*, was key."

WHERE DO THESE RULES COME FROM?

Let's take some time to think about the origins of these rules. As human beings, we all have a basic need to feel competent, to connect with others and to be loved, and to feel safe. Some people know these experiences to be true in their life. Unfortunately, for others, they do not always feel this way. From an early age, you may have developed and become accustomed to negative beliefs about yourself, including "I am a failure," "I am unlovable," "I am not good enough," "I am not safe" or "I am worthless."

In CBT, these underlying beliefs (positive or negative) are called "core beliefs". Core beliefs tend to be strongly held, have emotional intensity attached to them, and have likely been around for a while. Your rules for living are a way of protecting you against these beliefs – to keep them from springing up. Core beliefs are experienced with differing degrees of conviction and intensity, and will impact people differently. Put simply, core beliefs are at the root of the rules and the subsequent thoughts that we develop.

For example, if you have a core belief that you are a failure, you might constantly strive for success in life, and set up rules such as "In order to be successful, I must meet others' expectations of me at all times." This might later develop into a rule more specific to your eating problem, such as "In order to be successful, I need to be acceptable and attractive to others."

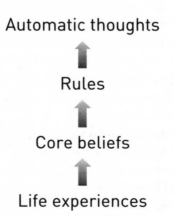

Automatic thoughts

⬆

Rules

⬆

Core beliefs

⬆

Life experiences

Let's tell you some more about Clare. Clare experienced high levels of criticism (weight related and general) as a young girl, and developed a belief that she was not good enough. She guarded against the fear that she was inadequate by pleasing others and trying to meet their expectations in order to feel successful. Clare developed a rule that others would think more positively of her if she was thin and if she demonstrated self-control over her eating. Left unchallenged, Clare's rule (which was developed as a young and vulnerable child) had remained fixed in her mind and she was still living by this rule ten years later. This meant she tried not to eat snacks and tried to control her food intake more generally. So, for Clare, what seemed like a simple (but overly strict) choice of not eating snacks had its basis in a rather powerful belief about herself. Unfortunately when these rules are too strict, they are unattainable. Inevitably you won't meet the mark, and the awful feelings of inadequacy that Clare feared would actually arise if she ate a snack. When, in fact, it wasn't really about the snacks at all!

IDENTIFYING YOUR CORE BELIEFS

Core beliefs can take more time to identify as they tend to be deep-rooted and perhaps less obvious. It is beyond the scope of this book to address core beliefs in great detail, but it can be helpful to understand the beliefs and fears that may be driving your eating problem.

One way of identifying the core of your problem is to continually ask yourself, "What is/would be the worst thing about that?" until you get to the root of it. For example, Clare thought about the situation with the snacks and the following internal dialogue occurred:

"You shouldn't have had that snack."

Q: What is the worst thing about that?

"Now you'll get fat."

Q: What would be the worst thing about that?

"People will judge me."

Q: What would be the worst thing about that?

"They'll see that I'm not good enough."

When we look at what underlies Clare's thoughts about eating the snacks, it is completely understandable why she felt so afraid.

To Clare, deep inside, snacking was equivalent to being thought of as inadequate. It wasn't really about the snack, but something far more entrenched.

It is vital to untangle the eating situations you struggle with from such important beliefs about yourself and the world, in order for things to feel different for you.

EXERCISE: IDENTIFYING YOUR CORE BELIEFS

Take some time to think about your own rules and beliefs:

Situation that caused me a difficult feeling (guilt, fear, shame, sadness):

What was the worst thing about this situation?

What would be the worst thing about that?

What would be the worst thing about that?

What do you believe that would say about you? About others? About the world?

SHIFTING CORE BELIEFS

Now you have identified your core beliefs, how do you shift them?

The best way to start is using the same strategies of looking at new ways of seeing things that we've already discussed. Bring these same approaches to the deeper underlying beliefs.

Clare wanted to foster a new belief that she *is* good enough. She looked for evidence on a daily basis that supported this belief rather than selectively attending to examples that she felt supported her "not good enough story". It is also important to act in a way that doesn't reinforce these beliefs, but challenges them. Rather than wait for the belief to change, act first. Our next chapter will talk about how you can challenge the way you *think* by what you *do*.

"Remind yourself that, as an adult, you have a chance to see yourself, others and the world differently. You don't have to continue to believe things you believed in the past."

Underlying core beliefs will take longer to change and may be attached to early, possibly painful, experiences. If this is the case, and these experiences and beliefs are at the root of your eating problem, then you might like to seek out the help of a face-to-face therapist in addressing these issues.

For now, remind yourself that, as an adult, you have a chance to see yourself, others and the world differently. You don't have to continue to believe things you believed in the past. You don't have to continue to live by the rules you developed at that time. You can choose to tell yourself that this is outdated, lacking in proof and will only be hurtful to you. Ask yourself now, how you would live if you could? What new, updated beliefs and rules would you like to live by from this moment on?

As Clare looked back on her childhood experiences of criticism, she could understand that her young self developed a belief that she was not good enough. As an adult, she realised that this was a misinterpretation, that she didn't deserve this level of criticism and that she *was* good enough. She felt sad for her younger self and realised she wanted to let go of this misunderstanding that she had been carrying with her all this time. She also then realised that this core belief was underlying her negative relationship with food. She decided to take charge and change her journey. She committed to practise a new guideline in her life – that it is okay to eat a full range of food with others. She was also determined to remind herself that she is good enough.

We have looked at identifying our unhelpful rules and beliefs that drive our pattern of thinking, and hopefully provided some tools to get started on challenging these. However, one of the most powerful ways to challenge thoughts, rules and beliefs is through acting differently. Often we wait until the conditions feel right before we change our behaviour; however, we want to encourage you to act first. Read on to find out how.

CHAPTER 14

FACING YOUR FEARS

There is another vital step to overcoming your eating problem. Not only is it important to challenge your thinking, we also need to test our thoughts with new behaviours. This is probably the hardest part of recovery, but also the most effective.

We understand that some of things we suggest in this chapter will contradict your natural inclination to stay away from situations that are associated with fear, guilt or shame. However, for your long-term health, we are going to challenge you to do the opposite! Keep reading below to see why and how.

STUCK IN THE SAME CYCLICAL PATH

As we have explored, you are caught up in your problem eating cycle for a good reason. The behaviours develop out of an attempt to cope with a difficult thought or feeling, or an effort to achieve something. So, what keeps these behaviours going?

AVOIDANCE

When we are afraid of something and we try (or are forced) to face it, we often find ourselves thinking of the worst-case scenario, worry that we won't cope and start to feel anxious and worried. Public speaking is a perfect example for many people. In that situation, it's not surprising we think how to escape the situation or stop it from happening. So, we pull away from what is making us feel uncomfortable. Avoidance is a very intrinsic human reaction to fear!

The problem with avoidance is that we never get to see what really happens if we face the situation. Essentially, avoidance builds a wall around you. It might make you feel safer, but it also makes your life more restricted and less free. One of life's challenges is to find ways to respond to these natural fears that help us grow and have the life we want to live, rather than staying stuck in a cycle of fear and avoidance.

UNHELPFUL COPING STRATEGIES

In addition to avoidance, you might use a variety of coping behaviours to keep the associated anxiety at bay. Broadly speaking, these unhelpful coping strategies allow you to face the fear, but *only* if you can use your way of making the situation less scary. In the instance of public speaking, you might make your speech, but avoid eye contact the whole time as a way of coping with your anxiety. Like avoidance, the problem with these behaviours is you don't truly face the underlying fear and you will never learn that people might be genuinely interested in what you are saying. You can become reliant on these behaviours to cope, but we want to help you think and act otherwise.

> "Avoidance is a very intrinsic human reaction to fear! The problem with avoidance is that we never get to see what really happens if we face the situation."

THE PROBLEM WITH THESE STRATEGIES

When we rely on avoidance or these coping behaviours, our fear never leaves. In fact, the more you rely on your avoidance or other behaviours to cope with your fears, the more likely you are to become stuck with them.

The behaviours you use, whether it's avoiding certain foods or restaurants, focusing on thinness, weighing yourself repeatedly or bingeing to avoid emotions, have no doubt made you feel better in the short term. That's why you keep using them. Perhaps they have worked to manage the unwanted feelings you experience around food. Perhaps they have given you an illusion of weight loss, or a sensation of feeling empty. Or maybe they help you feel in control. You now think that the only reason a terrible outcome hasn't occurred is because you avoided the situation or relied on your coping strategy.

Check out the below graph which depicts what happens when we avoid or employ unhelpful coping strategies. Notice how the fear keeps coming back time and time again, and to the same degree. What's more - we never get a chance to learn that fear passes. Once we learn to face our fears and sit with the anxiety, our fear response to a situation will reduce as we will realise there is no need to be afraid.

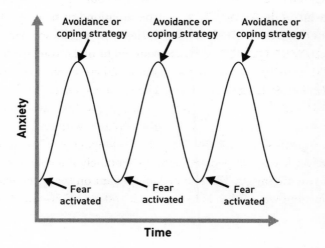

Have a look at the table below and see if any of these common behaviours apply to you:

FEAR	AVOIDANCE/COPING BEHAVIOUR
Fear of weight gain	Weighing yourself daily to ensure you haven't gained weight; calorie counting; avoiding carbs
Fear of losing control of eating	Following a rigid, strict meal plan, and not eating outside of this
Fear of others' judgement about appearance	Constantly comparing yourself to others
Fear of feeling full	Using compensatory behaviours to avoid this feeling
Fear of not being the slimmest	Never eating more than a friend
Fear of not managing emotions	Binge eating to avoid experiencing this emotion
Fear of eating in a certain restaurant	Avoiding these restaurants at the expense of seeing your friends

Let's now come back to Suki. She holds the belief that people will judge her body and not like her unless she loses weight. When faced with an invitation to a summer party, and knowing she needed to wear a cocktail dress, Suki felt self-conscious and anxious about her body. Her tendency in this situation is to use avoidance or an unhelpful coping strategy, as shown below.

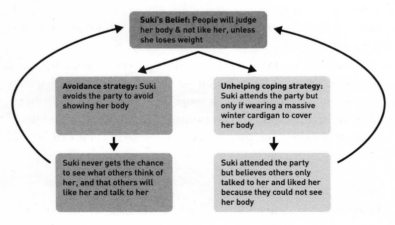

TRYING A NEW PATH

It is common for people with eating problems to want to change how they think and feel about food, eating and body image, but be more hesitant about behaviour change. We get this – it is really hard and can be scary to change.

Nonetheless, some fears and beliefs call for a dose of open-minded bravery. They call for intentionally facing your fears to shift your thinking.

For example, would you *really* gain weight if you ate pizza with your friends on Friday night? Would your friends *really* judge

"In order to overcome problem eating, you will ultimately need to take a plunge and experiment with the things you're afraid of, even when you're still feeling afraid or uncertain."

you if you chose what you actually wanted to eat rather than the low-calorie option? Would you *really* be out of control of your emotions if you didn't binge? As they say, there's only one way to find out...

We need to lean into the things we fear, and not escape before we have a chance to see what happens. In order to overcome problem eating, you will ultimately need to take a plunge and experiment with the things you're afraid of, *even when* you're still feeling afraid or uncertain. You can work to reassure yourself and prepare, but you can't wait until you don't feel afraid anymore. It is a case of "feeling the fear and doing it anyway".

If we continue to see a situation through, our feared outcome often doesn't occur. By slowly but surely facing the things that lead you to feel anxious or worried, you will gather new information to build accurate beliefs. Also over time, if you continue to face the things that worry you, you will feel less afraid. It will get easier.

HOW TO FIND A NEW WAY

Imagine for a moment that you are a therapist and you are treating a client with a phobia of dogs. They have a thought and a visual image of being attacked whenever they walk past a dog, with a strong feeling that this will definitely happen. Your client is completely avoiding dogs and any situation where a dog might be, to prevent themselves from feeling anxious. Your client is miserable because they really want to be able to go to the park, and to visit their dog-owner friends. If your client was asking your advice, what would you encourage them to do?

We imagine that you are thinking you might talk with them about their fear, encourage them to use some anxiety-management techniques, maybe talk to them about dogs, or show them some videos or pictures of dogs. However, before long, you would likely introduce the idea that the only way to overcome their fear was to face a real-life dog.

Now, you would probably not completely overwhelm them with a room full of Rottweilers! But you would probably start with a small dog from a distance, and build up to facing a dog at a closer and closer proximity. The more you face the dog, the more your anxiety will decrease over time. Why? Because you will get *corrective evidence* that, on balance, a dog is nothing to be worried about and that the chances of being attacked by a dog in the park are *extremely low*. That is, you'll find out what *really* happens when faced with a dog – and this information will help to *correct* your understandable but misguided fear. Let's come back to Suki.

When Suki realised how stressed the summer party made her, she felt fed up. She did not want her life to be dictated by the thoughts in her head. She didn't want to hide away any longer. After reflection, she realised that she cannot mind read and that people come in different shapes and sizes. She came up with an evidence-based alternative: "I may not want to wear a summer dress as I feel exposed, but I am sure others will be happy I am there and more focused on having fun." Suki needed to invest time into this thought and then let the old way of thinking go.

Suki *actually* wearing the summer dress without a baggy cardigan was *critical* to shifting the fear of others' judgement and supporting the new belief that others would just be happy that she was at the party. Unsurprising to us, she had a lot of fun.

Her friends all commented on how nice it was to see her finally join them, and how they really liked her outfit as well. From then on, Suki had to keep reminding herself of this truth. Of course, it didn't happen overnight, but eventually she noticed her old thoughts were definitely less frequent and certainly less powerful.

Sometimes, facing your fears once is enough to help you see things differently. If so, that's great! Often, though, you will need to face your fears many times over for the situation to gradually get easier. Research shows that this is what happens when we harness our bravery and *repeatedly* face our fears:

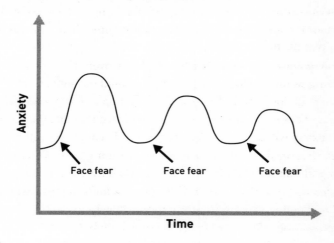

EXERCISE: PLAN YOUR OWN EXPERIMENT

Now is your opportunity to experiment with a new way of doing things that takes you away from your eating problems. You need to think about some ways that test out your negative thoughts and predictions you have about certain situations. That is, set up an experiment.

Remember the mantra, "Just because we think it, doesn't make it true"? Well, we need evidence to back up our new thought, and a behavioural experiment is your way of gathering that evidence.

It may be that you think going out for pizza with a friend will make you feel sick and that you won't manage the guilt, or that stopping weighing yourself on a daily basis will make your weight skyrocket, or that not wearing that certain item of clothing which hides your shape will mean people will comment on your weight. Have a think of a negative thought/prediction that drives a behaviour of yours, and one that you want to test out.

1. What is the thought or prediction that you would like to test out?
    For example: People at the party won't talk to me because they will judge me on my weight.

2. What is an alternative thought or prediction for this scenario? You might like to base this prediction on earlier work you have done on developing more balanced alternative thoughts.
    For example: People will talk to me at the party. They will like me with my body as it is.

3. Think about how you will test out the original prediction (in box 1). Plan the experiment in great detail.
   For example: I will go to the party as planned. I won't cover my body up. I will make effort to chat with people who talk to me.

4. Review the outcome. What happened? What do you conclude from the experiment? Do you need to adapt the experiment and try again?

COMMON BEHAVIOURAL EXPERIMENTS FOR OVERCOMING AN EATING PROBLEM

EXPERIMENT	FEARED OUTCOME THIS EXPERIMENT HELPS TO TEST OUT
Introducing avoided foods gradually	Do I gain loads of weight or lose control over my eating? (Note: in this scenario try to introduce previously banned foods slowly, and not when you're already hungry!)
Fears about weight/shape changes if you eat regularly	Does my weight skyrocket? (Note: you will need to weigh yourself no more than once weekly to test this fear out)
New eating-related situations e.g. a buffet	Do people judge me for eating at this restaurant?
Body image anxiety e.g. wearing tighter fitting clothes	Do people stare at me and avoid talking with me?
Responding differently to emotions	Do my emotions overwhelm me and do I lose control?
Communicating directly and clearly with others	If I say no, or express my own wishes/needs, am I rejected?
Fears about not meeting expectations	If I do my best and leave work on time, do I fail at work?

CREATING A NEW BEHAVIOUR IS HARD

Like a hiking trail, we are always more drawn to the well-trodden path that is familiar and well-practiced. We slip back into those ways easily. However, the more we practise alternative, more helpful behaviours, the more well-trodden this new path becomes. Keep it up!

As you practise, here are a few tips that might help along the way:

"Change is scary, particularly when you are really anxious about the outcome. We would recommend that you do not wait until you are less anxious to take these steps towards change."

- Tell someone supporting you what you're planning to do. Get them to help keep you accountable, and to be there for you while you face a fear.
- Prepare some strategies for coping if you get nervous.
- Have some encouraging statements ready.
- Practise taking some deep breaths.
- Visualise yourself trying out this new behaviour. That way, when you carry it out, it doesn't feel quite so "new".
- If it doesn't go to plan, speak to someone. Review what happened with an open mind. Could something have been done differently to give the experiment a greater chance of success?
- Remember you can learn and adjust from each new experiment. Keep going!

Change is scary, particularly when you are really anxious about the outcome. We would recommend that you do not wait until you are less anxious to take these steps towards change. In our experience, the fear is very often worse than the reality. As with everything, practice makes perfect so keep going even if you feel afraid.

Sometimes however, even when you have experimented and you know that your thinking is not accurate, the thoughts will continue. We have some ideas for these thoughts in the next section.

CHAPTER 15

WHEN THOUGHTS REMAIN STUCK

By now, we hope that some of the thinking techniques we have introduced make good sense and that you have given them a go. We also hope that you have noticed some beneficial effects from looking at your thoughts, evaluating their accuracy and usefulness, and started to practise telling your mind evidence-based alternative thoughts instead. You may have even set up some experiments to test it all out. If so, that's great.

"Your thoughts are like a well-trodden path; they are habitual and you can easily fall back into them."

However, as we have discussed, this takes time. Your thoughts are like a well-trodden path; they are habitual and you can easily fall back into them.

You might be reading this and thinking, "But I have tried all of this and my thoughts still feel stuck." You might have accepted that your thoughts are unhelpful and probably inaccurate, that you are engaging in various unhelpful thinking styles, and have spent time challenging thoughts throughout the day. You may be even giving the alternative thinking a good shot. However, some people still find themselves going over the same thought even when they *know* it's not true.

Maybe you review scenarios from the day, going over and over them, obsessing over every detail, worrying about what you ate, how you looked, or maybe what someone said to you/you said to someone else. Alternatively, you might be overly focused on thinking about the future and find yourself lost in thoughts about what is going to happen, planning what to wear on your upcoming beach holiday, what you will eat at your cousin's wedding and rolling through every case scenario in your mind. This is what we call "overthinking" – obsessing over things and having a thought go around and around your mind.

It is a normal part of life to reflect on our day, especially if we feel worried or sad about something, if we feel that we need to repair a relationship or to plan for the future in order to ensure a positive outcome. However, when these reflections become circular, and when the thoughts are no longer about finding a solution or finding the truth, then this becomes a problem.

"The problem with overthinking is this: it is not problem solving."

Overthinking is different to everyday reflections as it tends to take a lot of time and energy, and can be quite distressing. It is associated with anxiety, stress and low mood. It's also exhausting and doesn't really get us anywhere!

The problem with overthinking is this: it is not problem solving. Spending two minutes or 100 minutes thinking in a circular, problem-focused way will not bring you any closer to a solution. Not to mention, overthinking disconnects you from the here and now, the only moment in time when you have some control. This process of overthinking is much like a hamster running on a wheel: it takes a lot of time and energy, but it never gets far.

Let's look at Chris's overthinking for a moment. Chris had been struggling most days with a recurrent negative thought that "People think I'm greedy." This was usually triggered when he was eating his lunch at work. He had worked through the strategies we have covered in earlier chapters and identified that this thought was at the root of his distress. He had looked at the evidence and noted that 1) he did not know what others thought, 2) that people eat for survival and 3) that is not a typical conclusion to evaluate someone as greedy for having their sandwich and crisps at work. He could identify some of his unhelpful thinking styles: catastrophising, mind reading and jumping to conclusions. On balance, he concluded that the thought was irrational and decided to practise a more helpful thought, that "Eating my lunch is not greedy and if people think it is then they are looking at my eating with abnormal curiosity!" He had even carried out some behavioural experiments and practised more helpful alternative thoughts, noticing that people still didn't seem to comment or notice no matter what he ate at lunchtime!

However… Chris could still not shake this thought that others were thinking he was greedy. It had become a regular worry rather than just a thought. Not only that, but Chris would also get stuck worrying about *why* he was still worrying about this! He began judging himself for judging himself too! All this, unsurprisingly, made his overthinking even worse.

EXERCISE: YOUR STUCK THOUGHTS

Just for a moment, have a go at reflecting on the thoughts that get stuck in *your* mind — those which you tend to go over and over. Perhaps they are thoughts you *know* are irrational but just keep coming up all the time regardless. You may have talked with a friend about these thoughts to get reassurance and they have confirmed that they are unfounded, but they are still on your mind.

People tend to have various themes to their thoughts. It might be that you overthink about upsetting others, overthink calories, overthink your body shape, or overthink your performance at work. List them here, both the thoughts and the times these are most likely to be triggered.

Writing this down will help you be more aware of the repetitive thoughts to keep an eye out for, so you can notice when you are getting stuck.

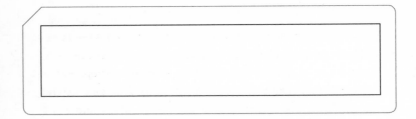

PATHWAYS AWAY FROM OVERTHINKING

PROBLEM-SOLVING

It is unlikely that you will be able to solve or to change anything by overthinking, especially if this involves the past or the future. However, finding a solution is often what people are trying to achieve by repeatedly thinking about something. Unfortunately, not all of life's problems can be solved. But some *can* be. If this is the case, then set aside some time to problem-solve in a structured and contained way. Shift your focus to the solution rather than the problem.

We are sure many of you will have your own ways of problem-solving as we all encounter cross-roads and decision points in life. Use the skills you already possess to help with the problems you are dwelling on.

EXERCISE: PROBLEM-SOLVING

You can also use the structured way of problem-solving below as another tool. Writing things down gives clarity of mind, and coming to a problem with an open mind gives you the best chance of finding the best solution for you.

- What is the problem? (Define clearly)
- What are the possible solutions? (List all)
- What are the pros and cons of each possible solution?
- Based on the above, what conclusion or decision have I come to?
- How can I implement this solution?

Once you've gone through this process, you might like to keep a copy of the conclusions you drew, nearby. Put a note on your phone or place a Post-It note in a location where you find yourself overthinking (e.g. on the bedside cabinet if you tend to do this before sleep). Let this remind you that you don't need to return to this problem, as you have already worked through it and decided on a course of action.

BEING MINDFUL OF OVERTHINKING

One of the first steps to overcoming overthinking is to notice the *process* of overthinking, rather than just the *content* of your over-thinking (i.e. the thoughts).

Mindfulness is the practice of being in the moment and is an useful way of managing the process of overthinking. It is a process of allowing thoughts to come and go without judgement. Mindfulness will help you identify when you are stuck in repetitive thoughts or when you are "on the hamster wheel again". It will allow you to step out of autopilot mode and into mindful mode to get some distance from your thinking, rather than feeling completely ruled by or enmeshed with your thoughts. Being mindful of your current experience involves noticing your thoughts and letting them pass. It is a way of reminding yourself that this "is just my mind having those thoughts again", and that you are more than just those thoughts.

Various metaphors have been suggested to help think about mindfulness of thoughts, for example observing our thoughts as though they are leaves passing by on a stream, items on a grocery store conveyer belt, clouds in the sky or even bullies on a bus[7]. The common thread is this: the thoughts/feelings/urges are just *part* of a picture rather than the whole picture, and *they pass.*

---

[7]   Harris, R. (2009). *ACT Made Simple: An Easy-To-Read Primer on Acceptance and Commitment Therapy.* New Harbinger: Oakland, CA, US.

SHIFTING YOUR ATTENTION

Another way to manage stuck thoughts is to build the "attention-shifting muscle" in your brain. When you notice that you are in an overthinking cycle, shifting your attention from inwards to outwards can help. This forces your mind to reduce its focus on the subject of the overthinking, and onto a neutral or pleasant object which is less threatening or less upsetting for you.

Some ideas for practising attention shifting are noticing what you see on your daily bus journey, or tuning into the various sounds as you walk down a busy street. Try to choose something non-threatening, making sure it is neutral or positive, and external to yourself.

EXERCISE: ATTENTION SHIFTING

1. Spend a minute allowing your mind to think about the particular negative thought that you feel stuck with or that you dwell on. For your first practice, you might want to choose a negative thought that is semi-distressing but not highly distressing. Make sure you only do this for one minute!

2. When a minute is up, find an object or a detailed (but non-threatening) picture to focus on for a moment.

3. Once you have chosen this object or picture, spend another minute looking at and describing to yourself all the detail – shapes, colours and size. There might be something around you in your environment you can focus on, or you might want to bring up a photo on your phone that is interesting and calming, such as a mountain scene.

4. What did you notice while doing this exercise? Did you find it easy to shift attention? Or is this something to keep practising?

After doing this task people often describe forgetting about the thought that was upsetting them, even momentarily, and often don't feel as anxious. Paying too much attention to your unhelpful thoughts will make them seem larger in your mind. When, in actual fact, nothing has changed – only the amount of time you have focused on it.

If you found that you could not shift your attention away, don't worry; this is common and normal when you first start to practise attention-shifting. Think of it as a muscle that takes time to build. You may want to start with the less "sticky" thoughts at first while you're building the muscle up to full strength. Keep heart though – with practise you will get there.

DISTRACTION

Sometimes you may need to shift your attention to a really distracting activity to help get you unstuck. This might be talking to a friend with whom you can have a really in-depth conversation, or it might be playing a game on your phone that takes all your concentration.

It is possible to become over-reliant on distraction and for this to become an avoidance strategy, keeping you away from paying attention to important things. However, unless you are overly relying on this technique, distraction does not need to be a process of avoiding or suppressing your thoughts. It can be a useful tool to refocus your attention away from your thought in the short term, when you are caught in an unhelpful overthinking process. You can then choose to go back and look at the content of your thought at a time that suits, or you can remind yourself that you've already problem-solved and you don't need to keep re-hashing it!

We find that often people use problematic eating behaviours (such as focusing on a diet, or binge eating) to distract themselves from emotions and from repetitive thoughts. If this is you, make a list of healthy distractions that leave you feeling good. See if you can choose something that is both distracting and one or more of the following: enjoyable, gives you a sense of achievement, or gives you a feeling of connection with others. These are the things that are known to improve mood, so you can also use distraction for your greater good!

CHANGE YOUR LOCATION AND GET MOVING

Another way to shift your attention is by actually getting up, out, and moving. Head out for a walk in nature, or see a friend. It does not need to be strenuous (although that can help), just something that will force your body to focus elsewhere. Try to leave your environment and remind yourself that another five minutes of thinking about whatever is worrying you will probably not get you any closer to a resolution or a sense of calm. Remember: it is the process of overthinking itself that is increasing your sense of being unsettled and worried.

"Remember: it is the process of overthinking itself that is increasing your sense of being unsettled and worried."

POSTPONE TILL LATER

For some people, the idea of setting aside a particular time dedicated to "overthinking" really works. To do this, set yourself a time in the day that you book in for yourself to think about the things that are really worrying you. We would recommend no more than half an hour for this. If you don't need the whole period of time you set aside, then just stop for the day – don't force yourself to keep going over things! During this time slot, you can think about what is on your mind in as much detail as you like and let your overthinking run amok. Once that time slot is up though, your overthinking also needs to be up.

Because overthinking often happens when we get "caught" worrying about a particular topic, we sometimes find that when the allocated time to overthink comes, there is nothing to worry about! All throughout the day if we've practised the process of "letting go" rather than "clinging on" when a repetitive thought comes into mind, the need for worry is likely to feel less.

> "Our thoughts become less stuck when we don't attend to them immediately."

The strategies we have outlined can be used when repetitive thoughts that are probably not true or helpful continue to enter your mind. Trying to get distance from these repetitive thoughts is key. Our thoughts become less stuck when we don't attend to them immediately. In a similar way, in order to get some distance from the distressing emotions we experience, we can learn to notice and observe them. More on that in the next chapter.

CHAPTER 16

DEALING WITH EMOTIONS

Many people are overwhelmed by their emotions and don't want to confront them. If this sounds like you, don't worry; this can be a normal response. However, confronting emotions is an important step towards managing eating problems, and we want to help you to understand why you have emotions and how to deal with them.

At this particular time in your life, having picked up this book, you could be experiencing more difficulty with emotions than usual. It might be that during the process of overcoming your eating problem, you will experience a variety of emotions. This can initially feel emotionally harder before it feels easier. If this is the case, keep going! Your emotions are probably signalling something that needs to be attended to. As you will see in this chapter, there are a lot of ways you can support yourself as these emotions arise. We want to give you some ideas for how you can acknowledge an emotion and handle it in a healthy way.

WHY DO WE HAVE EMOTIONS?

Emotions might be something you embrace, fear or that you are not particularly aware of day to day. They can be seen as something wonderful, something terrifying, or even as a sign of weakness. Whichever is the case for you, know that we all have emotions and experience a range of them on a daily basis. This is all part of being human.

Emotions play an important role in our survival. They "flag" desires and problems to us. They help inform us of things we want or need to change, via unpleasant emotions such as fear or disgust. They also help inform us of things we want and need to nurture, via pleasant emotions such as love and joy. Sometimes emotions even inform us of issues we had not been aware of on a thinking level. They also motivate our actions and decisions; for example, feeling anxious in preparation for an exam leads us to revise, feeling sad after a loss leads us to lie low for a time to grieve, and feeling empathy helps us connect to people in our life and support them when needed, thereby strengthening our relationships. We are social creatures and have always been a part of community. Our emotions are a way to communicate with our fellow human beings. They allow for greater warmth, intimacy and care.

> "Emotions are helpful indicators to us and communicators to others."

Put simply, emotions are helpful indicators to us and communicators to others.

Despite all of these important functions, for many people, and maybe for you, noticing, thinking about and expressing emotions can be painful and difficult.

WHERE DO WE GET OUR IDEAS ABOUT EMOTIONS?

Our early experiences shape us in many ways – our relationship with emotion being one of these. As a child, if your caregiver acknowledged and validated your emotions, and you were shown ways to respond to them, then you have likely learned that they're okay and can be managed. However, if your emotions were minimized, dismissed or discouraged, then they may be harder to experience and discuss now. Validation and helping a child to know what they are feeling teaches them that emotions are safe, acceptable and understandable – whether they are pleasant or unpleasant.

The way we witnessed our parents or caregivers handle their *own* emotions also impacts us. Seeing a caregiver experience an emotion, and use helpful and adaptive ways to cope with it, is a powerful learning point for a child. If you did not see this process, you may not have learned that emotions can be welcomed and dealt with in a healthy way. You may also have developed the misguided idea that emotions are *not* a part of normal healthy life. Alternatively, you may have witnessed emotion being dealt with using unhelpful coping strategies, such as self-criticism, food or alcohol, or angry outbursts. This can make emotions seem weak, frightening or even dangerous from a young age.

Have a think about how emotions were expressed, discussed, managed, validated or invalidated in your family. Then take a look at some common myths that develop out of these experiences below, and see if any apply to you.

COMMON MYTHS ABOUT EMOTIONS

- Emotions are a sign of weakness
- I won't be able to cope with my emotions
- If I let myself feel emotions, they will become out of control
- If I show my emotions, others will think I am mad or weak
- I should be able to cope with my emotions without support
- I shouldn't "give in" to negative feelings
- It is unacceptable to show emotions
- Emotions are a waste of time
- If I feel something, it must be true
- I shouldn't feel differently from others in a situation

SUPPRESSING OR NUMBING EMOTIONS

We often find that eating problems are linked to a pattern of suppressing or blocking emotions that feel overwhelming. This may numb or allow you to avoid the emotion, but the effects are short-lived. It also leads to a whole host of other problems and emotions for us to manage.

When you suppress or block emotions, they don't go away altogether. Instead, the emotion will just continue to bubble away until one day it comes out unexpectedly. This might reinforce your belief that emotions are out of control or dangerous, when in fact it was the *suppression* of emotion that contributed to the sense of being out of control, rather than the emotion itself. Moreover, expending so much energy on suppressing emotions actually prevents you from looking at the underlying issue and practising more helpful problem-solving skills.

In essence:

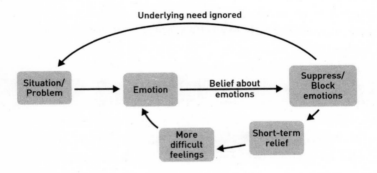

We understand that emotions can be unpleasant and that the temptation to avoid or numb them at all costs is often strong.

> "Trying to avoid the emotion will also postpone this crucial learning point: that *the intensity of emotion will pass.*"

However, trying to avoid the emotion will also postpone this crucial learning point: that *the intensity of emotion will pass.* Leaning into emotions and learning to accept them is an important part of life. If you do this, you will experience for yourself that intense emotion will pass. It has to. Your body simply cannot sustain that level of emotion forever. By using unhelpful ways to manage the emotion, you will be less equipped to tolerate the emotion and less likely to master more effective tools for coping.

Try instead to notice your emotion, lean into it, and be curious about what it is signalling. Then take care of yourself with compassion and warmth, as you allow it to pass. Read on for more about how to do this.

NOTICE YOUR UNHELPFUL WAYS OF MANAGING EMOTIONS

So, what do *you* currently do to cope? What are the strategies that you use? How do these help or hinder your eating problem?

Let's look at Suki for a moment. She identified that her binge eating often occurred after work when she felt anxious and stressed – often overthinking the challenging conversations she had with her colleagues during the day. Binge eating served the function of stress relief and temporary escape from anxiety. After a binge, however, not only did Suki feel uncomfortably full, she also felt shame, embarrassment, regret and guilt. Moreover, the anxiety and work stress felt worse, and Suki was stuck not knowing or experiencing how to *effectively* manage those emotions – so the cycle was set only to continue.

Let us be clear: enjoying food at the end of a busy day isn't the problem here. Food is pleasurable and we look forward to it. The problem is that Suki used binge eating to cope with her anxiety and had become over-reliant on food as her only source of pleasure and way to feel good.

Binge eating is not the only unhelpful strategy people use to manage emotions. Other coping behaviours might include restricting your intake, using compensatory behaviours, problem drinking, using illicit drugs, gambling, self-harm, or other risk-taking behaviour. Perhaps your own strategies are more subtle but still problematic – for example, avoiding contact with others, excessive social media usage or obsessive reassurance-seeking. Whatever you do, take some time now to think about the impact of your emotion coping strategies. Ask yourself:

- What are the consequences of my coping strategies? (Note: think in terms of finances, relationships, physical and emotional health, leisure, spiritual.)
- How do I feel straight after engaging in the coping behaviour? What about after an hour? Or the next day?
- What am I missing out on by using this coping strategy?
- Are they strategies I would recommend to a loved one, such as a child, who was experiencing the same situational stress?
- How do I want things to be different?

If you think you want to manage your emotions differently, and more skilfully, read on.

SO, WHAT CAN YOU DO TO MANAGE EMOTIONS?

There are many ways to manage emotion. Here we outline a few of these strategies. As you try these or practise them more than you currently do, be patient and kind to yourself, get support from others, and don't give up!

IDENTIFYING EMOTIONS

Identifying and understanding the underlying emotion for you is a powerful step in making sense of your eating problems and also in recovery. Notice when and how your body and mind are telling you that you are feeling something. Think about the emotions you feel the most. Maybe it is fear and anxiety? Or perhaps sadness and grief? Or shame and guilt? As much as possible, try to develop an emotional language that conveys what you are experiencing. And use words that fit for you. See opposite for a variety of emotions to get you started.

EXERCISE: WHAT ARE YOU FEELING?

Here is a non-exhaustive list of various emotions. If you have trouble naming your emotions, circle the ones you feel most readily.

Irritated	Fatigued
Sad	Serene
Happy	Surprised
Joyful	Self-assured
Hurt	Intimidated
Miserable	Excited
Ashamed	Trusting
Disgusted	Safe
Embarrassed	Proud
Distraught	Powerful
Ecstatic	Cautious
Guilty	Empathic
Fearful	Envious
Calm	Frustrated
Depressed	Alert
Worried	Powerful
Scared	Cheeky
Shy	Furious

GIVE YOUR BODY THE FUEL IT NEEDS TO MANAGE EMOTIONS

In order to manage our emotions, our body needs fuel. Regular nutrition throughout the day is therefore vital. Hungry people use food to manage feelings. Thinking of other healthier ways of coping will be harder if you are hungry.

"Hungry people use food to manage feelings. Thinking of other healthier ways of coping will be harder if you are hungry."

Even if you think that your eating problem is linked to emotions and not to dieting, it is absolutely vital to make sure your body has enough fuel to be able to think about managing your emotions effectively. This means eating regularly is a core emotion management strategy.

BUILD EMOTIONAL RESILIENCE

To manage emotions, we need to have energy. If the stress in our life outstrips the resources we have, we won't be able to do this. A good analogy here is to think about your emotional resilience levels fluctuating like water in a bucket. The bucket gets drained by the demands and stressors we face in life, and by chronic difficulties that slowly drain us. It gets topped up by things that rejuvenate us. When the balance is insufficient, you start to feel symptoms of burnout – such as exhaustion, difficulty concentrating, mood swings, difficulty sleeping, and anxiety. Somewhat like this example:

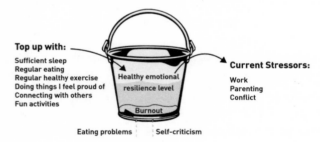

Top up with:
Sufficient sleep
Regular eating
Regular healthy exercise
Doing things I feel proud of
Connecting with others
Fun activities

Healthy emotional resilience level

Burnout

Current Stressors:
Work
Parenting
Conflict

Eating problems   Self-criticism

Often in our busy lives, we don't fully acknowledge the level of demand being placed on us. It's important to notice how much you are dealing with in order to understand why you are feeling the way you are. Sometimes, you might be over-committed or over-worked. If so, ask yourself: is there anything I can let go of at this time to keep my emotional resilience level in check?

Things that might help to "top up" resilience levels include caring for your body with regular sleep, regular nutrition and regular exercise. It also helps to routinely do things that make you feel good. Ask yourself: have I been doing enough of these things to give myself emotional energy? Is there anything else I could add in?

You might also like to think about whether there are any chronic "leaks" in your resilience bucket. For example, regularly criticizing yourself will slowly diminish your resources. In the same vein, so will a pattern of striving for perfection, of blaming yourself, or of pushing others away so you are not supported. Do you have any of these patterns that are slowly depleting your emotional resources?

CALM YOUR BODY

Use your breath to help regulate the impact of emotion in your body. This can be especially helpful if you are experiencing fear, agitation or irritability. If the emotion is accompanied by difficulty breathing, muscle tension, sweating, shaking, or a racing mind, then use breathing to release the tension you are feeling. To do this, try the following exercise:

EFFECTIVE BREATHING

Let's start with your breathing. Don't underestimate just how valuable effective breathing can be. Here is a breathing exercise to help you.

Count to four as you breathe in, then count to six as you breathe out. Close your eyes, clear your mind, and focus on your breathing. One of the first things that usually happens when you start to panic is that your breathing speeds up, so concentrating on exhaling for six seconds can help calm you down. The outward breath releases tension in the chest too. Don't forget to try this at home when you're already feeling quite calm and then practise it more and more so you can use it in increasingly stressful situations.

COMFORT YOURSELF

We are all born needing to be soothed and comforted. It's an evolutionary requirement. If we see a baby upset or unsettled, we are naturally drawn towards soothing them with our senses – for example, humming, singing, rocking them, dimming the lights, feeding them or stroking their head. These are all sensory activities.

As an adult, nothing changes. Our senses can still be used to comfort us when we feel upset or distressed. This is why using food to comfort ourselves during times of emotion can be a reinforcing activity, because it feels good and also soothes our senses.

We have discussed that food can be used for pleasure. However, we want to encourage you to find other ways to use your senses to comfort yourself. Have a look at the list below and think about what works for you, or develop your own list. We are all unique and find different things calming and comforting in moments of distress.

Sight – contemplating an ocean view, looking at old photos, watching a funny film, going to the local garden to see nature

Touch – using hand cream, getting a massage, stroking a pet, having a shower or bath

Smell – breathing in the smell of lavender, fresh lemon or freshly cut grass

Sounds – hearing ocean waves, rain on a tin roof, piano music (Tip: the Calm app has loads of different sounds to choose from)

Taste – drinking a nice cup of herbal tea, mindfully eating your favourite food

SHIFT YOUR FOCUS

Often, strong emotions are connected with our brain being lost in memories of the past, or worries about the future. So, connecting with the present moment is useful when you feel completely overwhelmed, or your mind is in a whirl of emotions and thoughts.

You could also try "grounding" yourself in the present by literally feeling the ground under your feet. Place your feet firmly on the floor and notice the feeling of being anchored. This is a safe and secure feeling. You can come to it any time you need.

CONNECT WITH THE PRESENT MOMENT

In a moment of stress, try the below:

- Name 5 things you can see.
- Name 4 things you can touch.
- Name 3 things you can hear.
- Name 2 things you can smell.
- Name 1 thing you can taste.

EXPRESS YOURSELF

Find an outlet or a way to express exactly how you feel. For some this is crying, or talking to others about how they feel, while for others creative expression works best. Many people find it difficult to discuss how they feel. They may know exactly *what* they are feeling, but the act of talking it out with someone can be really difficult. If this is you, first try journaling and just writing out on paper how you feel. Many people who prefer this medium of communication describe how cathartic it can be to "download" this information on paper. In addition to writing, perhaps you'd like to create something. Use the emotion to write songs, paint, sculpt — whatever works for you. As long as you are finding a way to express the emotion and have an outlet that is healthy to yourself and others, you are making progress.

TALK TO SOMEONE

Letting someone know how you feel can alleviate the pressure of sitting with the emotion. If a loved one knows that you struggle with intense emotions, or that a certain emotion can trigger self-destructive behaviour, then share that you are feeling that way. Perhaps suggest you do something together or find a way to distract yourself with their company. Again, it is important here to not let this strengthen the emotion. You want the loved one to recognize that the best thing will probably not be to overthink the situation, but to help support you to do something more helpful and interrupt the cycle of unhelpful behaviour. Remember, the emotion will pass. Being with someone will help this happen.

EMBRACE EMOTION

We have all experienced unpleasant emotion, and we have all experienced misfortune. Life can be difficult, and a variety of emotions are all part of being human. Accepting this human experience, rather than fighting it, can actually make us stronger. We are not proposing learned helplessness here, or the sense that we have no power over our situation. Quite the opposite. By making room for a variety of emotions, we can enable ourselves to not be so afraid of them, which gives these emotions less strength and control over us.

Making room for emotion, as well as using different ways of managing emotion, are important tools to change our relationship with our feelings. In the next chapter we discuss body image – a key feature for most people with eating problems – and one that also evokes a lot of strong feeling. Join us as we think about how you can tackle the distress and upset your body image might be causing you.

CHAPTER 17

BODY IMAGE

Body image is how we perceive, think and feel about our physical appearance, and can be a core aspect of eating problems. Sadly, body dissatisfaction is so common, even among people without eating problems, that it has been considered a normal dissatisfaction in our current society.[8] Despite increasing messages of body positivity, current shape and weight ideals continue to be promoted through the media and show no sign of changing. Let's be clear, body image is not just a female issue. There is increasing pressure on women and men to adhere to societal standards of attractiveness, which leads to body comparisons and body dissatisfaction. For people with eating problems, shape and weight control tends to be prized. Achieving a certain body shape, be it thinness, muscularity, or muscle tone, can become an all-consuming goal. As well as being highly valued, body size is often a central part of someone with an eating problem's identity and central to how they may evaluate themselves. So, what impacts body image, and what can we do about it?

WEIGHT BIAS

It goes without saying that in our current culture there is a bias towards a slim physique for women and a muscular physique for men. This is what we call weight bias. This therefore means

---

8   Rodin, J., Silberstein, L., & Striegel-Moore, R. (1984). Women and weight: A normative discontent. *Nebraska Symposium on Motivation, 32*, 267–307.

that being in a larger body is not desired, and not only that, that it is something to be ashamed of or that you should be striving to change. This leads to negative attitudes, beliefs and assumptions towards individuals who do not fit the "thin ideal". These negative weight-related attitudes, beliefs, assumptions and judgements towards size and weight have all sorts of negative effects on us and on society.

Societal weight bias comes from a misguided belief that higher weight is always related to poor health. You may have heard of the Body Mass Index (BMI). This was intended as a research tool, not a diagnostic tool, but is now involved in common clinical practice as a gauge of physical health. Although it can be useful when conducting research, in clinical practice it is a crude, stand-alone measure that doesn't consider someone's global health (physical, emotional, psychological, social, financial) or various age, sex and ethnic norms. Focusing solely on BMI at the exclusion of other health markers is problematic, and can contribute to weight stigma.

There is also evidence to show that weight stigma and bias might be causing some of the negative health outcomes often associated with being a higher weight, rather than weight (or BMI) itself. Unfortunately, many studies that look at the impact of "obesity" on health do not consider how weight stigma and weight bias could also potentially be contributing to these poorer health outcomes.

Some of the problems with which weight bias and stigma have been associated include:[9]

- Body dissatisfaction
- Low self-esteem and self-confidence
- Feelings of worthlessness and loneliness
- Suicidality

---

[9]   Alberga, A. S., Russell-Mayhew, S., von Ranson, K. M., & McLaren, L. (2016). *Weight bias: a call to action*. Journal of Eating Disorders, 4, 34.

- Psychiatric illness including depression and anxiety
- Over-eating and out-of-control eating
- Unhealthy eating patterns and eating disorders
- Avoidance of physical activity and lower motivation to exercise
- Stress-induced illness
- Avoidance of medical and health care

At its worst, repeated experiences of this weight bias from the media (print and social), family, friends, colleagues and even health professionals, can make you start to believe these messages are true. This is what we call an internalised weight bias.

An internalised weight bias doesn't need to be directly shaming. For example, the comment "Wow, you look great, have you lost weight?", although well intended, might inadvertently reinforce the belief that you are only valuable or worthy of praise if you are a certain weight or shape. This could be particularly problematic if someone has used unhealthy or extreme methods to get to this shape or weight, as it might make them more inclined to continue this unhealthy cycle.

Take a moment to have a think about whether you have your own internalised or externalised weight bias? If the answer is yes, this is not your fault! This is a product of our weight-centric culture, but now that you are aware of the consequences, it doesn't have to continue to be this way. What can you do to challenge your own weight bias?

FAT TALK

Weight bias/stigma can lead to "fat talk". Fat talk (or weight talk) is the language and words we use in conversation that can reinforce unhelpful prejudices about shape and weight. They can be employed in a bullying or shaming way, or more innocently and without malicious intent. However, in all cases, fat talk reinforces weight biases and is associated with increased body dissatisfaction.

Have a think about how often you notice yourself or others engaging in fat talk. You might find that this happens a lot in your day-to-day conversations. If so, we want to encourage you to find a way to disengage from these conversations to look after your body image and the body image of those you talk to.

WAYS TO AVOID 'FAT TALK'

- Make your home a fat-talk-free zone. Make a commitment with your family, partner or housemates to avoid fat talk.
- When commenting on others, try to highlight the positive parts of their personality, or the things about them that actually matter – not just their appearance!
- Think about and alter the wording you use to discuss body shape and appearance.
- If it feels too uncomfortable to challenge a friend or family member, try to divert the conversation instead.
- Think about an impressionable child. Perhaps imagine your child, your future children, your nieces/nephews, or a friend's child. Would you want them to pick up on fat talk?

THE ORIGINS OF YOUR BODY IMAGE

Much like our thinking style, the value we place on shape and weight comes from somewhere. Perhaps you have had painful experiences of being teased or marginalised because of your shape and weight. Maybe you have negative experiences of being taken to professionals as a child in order to lose weight. Or you are in a circle of friends that talks about weight all the time, count calories and highly value shape. Or, let's face it, you live in this current society where we are constantly being bombarded with misleading messages that thin = beautiful and thin = health.

EXERCISE: BODY IMAGE ORIGINS

Have a think about the factors, experiences or influences that have given rise to the value you place on shape and weight or your own weight bias.

Here is an example of Suki's ideas about what contributed to her body image.

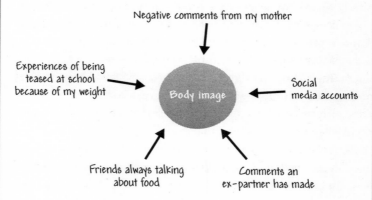

Now it's your turn. Brainstorm below what issues and experiences have contributed to your own body image:

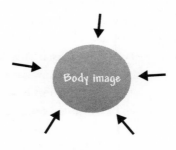

UNDERSTANDING YOUR BODY

Some body image problems come from a misunderstanding about what is happening as our body changes throughout the day. You might weigh yourself and panic when you see small fluctuations, thinking that it must mean your weight is shooting up. Maintaining your weight does not mean being the exact same weight every day of the week. Weight "maintenance" is actually when your weight settles within a *range* of few kilograms over a long period of time, with normal weight fluctuations occurring within this. Our weight actually fluctuates up to 1–2 kg throughout the day. This is normal and mainly due to fluid shifts in the body. Our weight fluctuates during the day and between days for a huge variety of reasons, including when we last ate and drank, when we last passed urine or opened our bowels, sweating, and a woman's menstrual cycle.

To make sense of long-term weight changes (changes in muscle and fat), we need to discount daily weight fluctuations. Weighing yourself no more than once a week will allow you to see any long-term pattern. Weighing yourself more frequently will mean that you only see the daily weight fluctuations, which could leave you feeling very anxious as you may misinterpret fluctuations as being a long-term weight change.

Our shape also changes after eating, with our stomach appearing full. Next time you eat and feel worried about changes in your body, ask yourself if you are mistaking something temporary for something permanent. The most common example of this is to mistake fullness for fatness. A changed stomach shape and a full feeling after eating are *not* the same things as weight gain.

"A changed stomach shape and a full feeling after eating are *not* the same things as weight gain."

CONTEXT MATTERS

You may find that you feel worse about your body when you are feeling worse in general. Low self-esteem and poor body image are closely related. Body image is not static and tends to fluctuate depending on your context. Some contextual factors that can impact how you are feeling about your body include tiredness, having just eaten, the time of day, or even what you are wearing (e.g. tight-fitting clothes). There are likely also times, places and situations that you tend to feel better about your body. For example when you're feeling relaxed and happy, when you're with friends who don't aren't body critical, when you're wearing an outfit you love.

A common time when body image can worsen, for women, is when she is on her period, as not only can hormones cause our mood to change, but normal, functional bloating can occur. In addition, people often discuss how certain environments can affect their body image – common examples include the beach, shopping malls or just being with friends who might be dressed differently to you. Remember in these moments that just because you are thinking negative thoughts about your body does not mean they are true – nor does it mean that your body needs to change.

"Just because you are thinking negative thoughts about your body does not mean they are true – nor does it mean that your body needs to change."

EXERCISE: SITUATIONS THAT IMPACT YOUR BODY IMAGE

Take some time to list the contexts or environments that are related to a worsening body image for you:

```
┌─────────────────────────────────────┐
│  ┌───────────────────────────────┐  │
│  │                               │  │
│  │                               │  │
│  │                               │  │
│  │                               │  │
│  └───────────────────────────────┘  │
│                                      │
│  Also take some time to list contexts or environments that are │
│  related to an improved body image for you:                    │
│                                      │
│  ┌───────────────────────────────┐  │
│  │                               │  │
│  │                               │  │
│  │                               │  │
│  │                               │  │
│  │                               │  │
│  └───────────────────────────────┘  │
└─────────────────────────────────────┘
```

YOU ARE MORE THAN YOUR BODY

Body image can become an all-consuming facet of how we view and feel about ourselves. Sadly this can take over and stop us from thinking about the other aspects of who we are as people, and about what it is really important to us in life. The exercise below aims to help keep body image in its rightful place, as just one aspect of who you are, by giving you time to think about what really matters to you.

EXERCISE: WHO YOU ADMIRE

For a moment, think of someone that you admire. It may be someone that you work with, a tutor at university or a family friend; someone from your present life or someone from the past. Now, write a list of their characteristics that you find admirable.

Who I admire:

Why I admire them:

Reflect on your list. What do you notice? How many characteristics are appearance- or shape- and weight-related?

Often when people do this task, they find that the things they value in others have little to do with their body shape and much more to do with their inner qualities – their character, strengths and values. You will probably also notice that what you value about others is more to do with who they *are* rather than how they *look*.

LIVING YOUR VALUES

Let's use some pie charts to think about weight and shape differently and return to the example of Clare.

Shape and weight are extremely important to Clare's identity and self-esteem. She has struggled with an obsession over her shape and weight for a long time, and feels miserable as a result. She is unable to enjoy herself when she is out because all she can think about is her body and worrying about what others are thinking of it. Clare finds herself obsessing about her shape because it matters so much to her.

Here is an example of a pie chart that depicts just how important Clare's shape and weight is currently, compared with other elements that make up her identity and self-esteem:

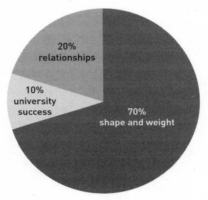

As you can see, 70% of Clare's identity and self-esteem is reliant on her shape and weight. However, there are so many other interesting and wonderful aspects of Clare that make up who she is as a person. When Clare really thinks about what she wants as the focus of her identity and self-esteem, she comes up with the below "ideal" pie chart:

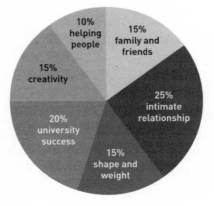

By using these pie charts, Clare could think about what was missing in her life and what she needed to devote more time to (e.g. creativity). This helped her move in the direction of her ideal pie chart. She made the commitment to enrol in an art class to enlarge her life. She also booked a night out with her boyfriend and forfeited one of her classes at the gym. The results for Clare were two-fold. She nurtured the focus on her relationship and on art that she wanted, and by doing so she had less time to focus on the shape and weight preoccupation she wanted to reduce.

EXERCISE: LIVING YOUR VALUED LIFE

Now it's your turn. First, make a list of the things in life that are currently important to how you view yourself. Things that contribute *right now* to my identity / self-esteem:

Don't worry if shape and weight are on the list. They are for a lot of people. Now decide how much importance you place on each of these aspects, by dividing the pie chart up accordingly.

Next, take some time to make another list of all the things that you want to give you meaning and worth as a person. Perhaps these are things that have been important to you but have taken a backseat lately, or they are areas of your personality and life you've always wanted to nurture but have never got around to.

Things that I want to contribute to my identity/self-esteem:

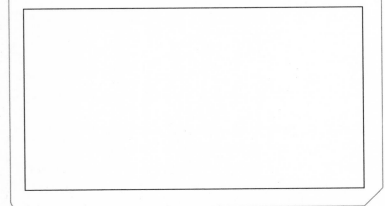

Finally, decide how much importance you want to place on each of these aspects, by dividing the pie chart up accordingly:

Take some time to reflect on your actual and ideal pie charts. What do you notice? What's different?

We challenge you now to make a commitment. What do you need to change in the here and now to get to the second pie chart and help you enlarge your life? What practical changes could you make this week?

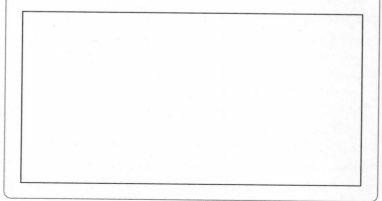

BE SOCIAL-MEDIA SAVVY

The rise of social media has created new challenges in the way we compare our bodies with others. Body comparisons tend to maintain our issues with shape and weight dissatisfaction.

Given the availability of photo-editing tools, and the capability to convey "perfect" (but wholly unrealistic) body shapes, it is important to be social-media savvy. Be mindful of the accounts you follow and whether or not these are really all that inspiring. If something makes you feel "less than", then delete it or unfollow it. Do it as an experiment and notice if unfollowing the account makes you feel better or worse. If you find that you are actively searching for these accounts or obsessing over them, give it some time and see if you are still obsessing in a couple of weeks.

Also think about the amount of time spent on social media. Perhaps, if this is an area that is particularly challenging for you, have a go at reducing your social media time or try out a digital detox. You might even want to experiment with having two days on and two days off social media, so you can truly see the difference. We find that few people (if any) ever regret making this change to their social media habits.

Here are some tips to wise up to socials:

- Have some social-media-free time a day and put limits on your phone to manage this.
- Remember that many photos are edited and airbrushed, therefore you are probably comparing yourself to something that isn't even real!
- Only follow accounts that inspire you and make you feel good, and bin those that make you feel "less than" or that trigger you. This also includes friends and family who post unhelpful content. If you don't want to delete their accounts, it may be helpful just to unfollow them so that they don't appear on your feed. Think about your pie chart exercise – who do you now want to follow?
- Beware of advertising. Social media is an online version of a

glossy mag. Be mindful of the subliminal messages trying to make you feel rubbish about yourself in order for a company to make money from women who feel dissatisfied or less than.

CHECKING AND AVOIDING

Sometimes people who are unhappy with their body cope with this feeling by checking their body constantly – for example, by looking in the mirror for long periods of time, repeatedly weighing themselves, measuring body parts obsessively, or poking and prodding their body looking for the "imperfections" they fear.

Others cope by avoiding their body. That is, not looking in the mirror, avoiding shop-window reflections, never wearing a swimming costume, or avoiding clothes that bring attention to their body.

Both checking and avoiding increase the chances of an inaccurate body image.

When you body-check, the attentional focus on shape and weight makes you more likely to overestimate any perceived flaws and build an inaccurate mental representation of your body. Take weighing for example. How many people, when trying to lose weight, find themselves religiously weighing themselves multiple times a day? By weighing yourself loads, you run the risk of misinterpreting and catastrophising over the small, and expected, weight fluctuations we discussed earlier. Similarly, it is not difficult to convince yourself that you have gained weight by touching and pinching your stomach after a roast dinner. But the belief that you have gained significant

"It is not difficult to convince yourself that you have gained weight by touching and pinching your stomach after a roast dinner. But the belief that you have gained significant weight after one meal is simply not accurate!"

weight after one meal is simply not accurate! Weight and shape temporarily change after eating, and this change will reverse again. Checking your body after eating is unhelpful.

On the other hand, if you avoid your body, you might not get valuable and corrective feedback about your body weight. Not to mention, you might not experience all the wonderful opportunities that your body affords you. You will be aware of some of your avoidance behaviours. Perhaps you dread wearing a swimming costume and avoid swimming as a result. Others you will be less aware of. Perhaps you are uncomfortable in photos but not really sure why. Is it possible you are avoiding seeing your image? Or perhaps you try not to sit too closely to people. Is it possible you are avoiding becoming aware of your body because intimacy feels scary?

We think challenging yourself to address these checking and avoidance behaviours is key to improving your body image. This will likely reduce the intensity and negativity of your thoughts and improve how you feel – if not in the short term, then definitely in the long run.

If you are finding it tough to change these behaviours, set small, achievable targets. If you are spending excessive amounts of time looking at yourself in the mirror, perhaps you can decide to gradually reduce this. Similarly, you could limit yourself to only weighing yourself once a week if you are compulsively weighing. Or, to be even more radical, ditch the scales altogether!

EXERCISE: WHAT CAN YOU CHANGE?

Have a think about your body checking and body avoidance behaviours. How can you change/reduce them over time?

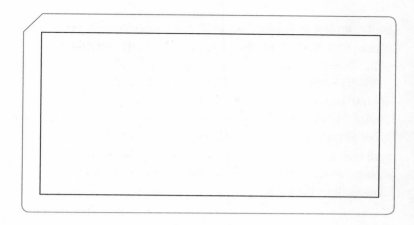

YOUR BODY IS AMAZING

An over-focus on the appearance of our body is a form of objectification. How do you feel when you see people being objectified? It's not nice, right? So why do we do this to *ourselves*? It's so easy to get caught with a focus on the appearance of our body – prodding and poking it as if it is an object. We think it's unlikely you would stand for it if you saw your friend being objectified in this way.

When we objectify our bodies, we don't tend to focus on the intricacies and scientific wonders of how our body works and what it does on a daily basis. Our body does so much to keep us alive, to help us enjoy life with others, and to help us achieve our goals.

Have a think about all of the amazing things that your body does for you. Try to come up with as many as you can and write them all down. Maybe even start to thank your body and make peace with it.

Check out Clare's list below.

- Listens to music
- Types on my computer
- Dances
- Takes photos

- Breathes
- Listens to a podcast
- Travels the world

Try to remind yourself of all of the things your body does for you over and above appearance. And remember, what you *do* with your body is more important than how it *looks*.

"Remember, what you do with your body is more important than how it *looks*."

Let's now look at mindfulness as another skill to help us be at peace with ourselves — including with our bodies and our relationship with food.

CHAPTER 18

THE PRACTICE OF MINDFULNESS

You may love or hate it when you hear the word "mindfulness", but we think it is so helpful in your journey towards managing problem eating. This is because being on autopilot is at the centre of so many eating problems. Mindfulness expert Jon Kabat-Zinn talks of mindfulness as a practice, rather than a tool or technique. This emphasises that mindfulness isn't something to be achieved or just a good idea, more so a way of being.[10]

The common misconception made about mindfulness or meditation is that it aims to clear the mind. It is therefore no wonder that many get frustrated that they are doing it "wrong", because this is an impossible task. Mindfulness is actually about awareness. It is about becoming aware in the moment of what is happening in your environment, body and mind – without judgement. It is a way of slowing things down and helping you get out of autopilot, so that you can simply observe what your mind is thinking, and what you are feeling or experiencing. By observing your experiences without judgement, and bringing a degree of acceptance and compassion to your current moment, it can result in you feeling less overwhelmed.

Mindfulness also allows us to notice that thoughts and feelings come and go. When we accept that the moment "is what it is" and don't expend energy trying to fight it, then we have a chance to spend that same energy on making choices about how to respond.

---

[10] Williams, M. & Penny, D. (2011). *Mindfulness: A practical guide to Finding Peace in a Frantic World*. Piatkus: London, UK.

For example, when Chris is emotionally eating, he is on autopilot. He is unaware of what he is eating and unaware of what's going on inside him that's driving him to keep eating. For Chris, his binges are preceded by feeling sad, and he uses eating to "zone out" and to distract himself from the sadness because it feels uncomfortable. Later, he feels worse. Practising mindfulness was helpful for Chris to overcome this cycle by increasing awareness of what was going on inside him – noticing emotional shifts, hearing what his body needed, and eating with mindful, conscious awareness of what he was consuming. It also helped him to realise that his sadness will pass.

"Mindfulness can be helpful in many different forms, but all draw on the *practice* of paying attention to the present moment."

GIVE IT A GO

Mindfulness can be helpful in many different forms, but all draw on the *practice* of paying attention to the present moment.

Let's start with an exercise to help with this practice.

EXERCISE: BEING MINDFUL

Right now, in this moment, try to focus fully on the here and now. Shift your focus outwards and engage your senses. Notice what you can see, what you hear, what you smell, and what you can touch. Try not to change or evaluate the situation; just become aware of what you notice. After some time, you may find that your mind starts to wander or it starts to put a story together about what you are noticing. Perhaps you wonder why the alarm in the distance has gone off, or you remember that you forgot to take the bins out, or you start planning what to have for dinner later. A wandering mind is normal – this is what minds do. Minds struggle to stay in the present and try to

---

move to the future or the past. When this happens, just notice it, without judging or chastising yourself, and just gently bring your attention back to the here and now.

It is really normal and common for this exercise to feel really difficult at first. Like many of the techniques in this book, it takes practice, practice, practice to bring a non-judgmental awareness to our experiences. Think of it like an under-developed muscle that needs strengthening. It's important to build this muscle as it helps us to be less reactive in life and to be more open to the full range of our human experiences. It also helps us to be understanding and kind to ourselves as human beings, because we practise noticing what brings us joy, what makes us sad, and what we need in life, all without judgement. So, it is definitely a muscle worth building!

MINDFUL EATING

You can also use mindfulness in your experience of eating. Mindful eating is often framed as "eating when you're hungry and stopping when you're full". However, this is not quite right. Mindful eating can easily be turned into the next diet to lose weight, which it is not. Mindful eating is not about trying to control how much you eat, but rather increasing awareness of why we eat, what happens when we eat, and increasing our enjoyment of food.

Mindful eating is bringing awareness to eating food in the present moment without any judgement. It allows us to have a natural experience with food and be reconnected to our senses while we eat. That is, how the food looks, what it sounds like, what it smells like, what it tastes like, what it feels like in our hands, in our mouth and as we eat it. It is noticing what is going on with curiosity, without trying to change anything about it.

BENEFITS OF MINDFUL EATING

Various benefits of mindful eating have been reported by the Center for Mindful Eating.[10] These include:

- Improvement in eating habits
- Improvement in lifestyle
- Reduction in body dissatisfaction
- Increased enjoyment with eating
- Improvement in psychological health, including anxiety, depression, self-esteem and quality of life
- Increased awareness of internal cues
- Increased awareness of why we choose food
- Decreased guilt attached to food and eating
- Decreased compulsive eating, emotional eating and comfort eating

In an effort to improve her relationship with food, Suki had been challenging herself by eating one of her fear foods – chocolate. She noticed that this challenge was proving difficult. She took a few moments to reflect on what was happening, and noticed a pattern of eating chocolate quickly while standing in the kitchen. She had read about mindful eating and thought she would give it a go.

When next eating chocolate, she decided to sit down at the dining table instead of standing in the kitchen. She took time to notice the colour of the wrapper. Normally she opened the chocolate quickly, but this time she noticed that the lettering was raised. She also noticed the noise it made as she moved the wrapper between her fingers.

Then Suki noticed the nutritional information jumping out at her from the wrapper. Her mind started calculating calories, and escalated quickly to thoughts of being greedy. Her heart started racing and her face became hot and flushed. Suki was able to notice this chain of events, and instead of continuing down this path by criticising herself, she stopped, took a deep breath, and went back to noticing the lettering on the wrapper. She opened the wrapper and broke off a piece, noticing the crack of the chocolate. She held it between two fingers and noticed how the heat of her body had started to soften it. She noticed the dark colour and how it had one perfectly straight side while the other was uneven. She brought the chocolate up to her nose and noticed the scent of cocoa. She put the square in her mouth and let it sit there melting, noticing the texture move from hard to soft. She closed her eyes and tried to describe the taste she was experiencing.

Her mind started to think about what else she ate that day and how she would compensate for this later, but she noticed this happening and, without judging herself, kindly brought herself back to the experience in her mouth and how it felt as she swallowed it.

Suki reflected on her experience afterwards and noticed that when she ate standing up in the kitchen, she didn't taste or experience the chocolate in any way. She always felt guilty afterwards, and this led her to try to compensate by eating a smaller dinner. When she tried to eat the chocolate mindfully, she noticed that she enjoyed not only the taste of the chocolate, but the texture. She noticed how much judgement she had attached to the chocolate and how quickly it had escalated to an unpleasant emotional and physical response. But, she also felt empowered that it brought an increased awareness as to why she had been eating it so quickly while standing in the kitchen, and why it led her to eat less at dinner and binge later in the evening. It was not just her hunger that was triggering the binge, but also that she had not allowed herself to enjoy the chocolate. She noticed that she may have also been punishing herself later by bingeing because of the feelings of guilt she had experienced but not recognised in the moment.

Through this practice, Suki noticed that she would initially berate herself for not being able to "do" mindfulness properly. She noticed herself having this self-judgement, and again drew her mind to the sensation of eating. Over time, through her mindfulness practice, she was able to slow things down, fully engage her senses while eating, and consequently noticed an improvement in her binge eating.

WHAT THINGS CAN YOU DO TO HELP YOU PRACTISE MINDFUL EATING?

- Focus on what the food and drink looks like, smells like, tastes like and how it feels in your mouth.
- Notice any judgments, and gently escort your attention back to the act of eating and drinking.
- Slow down eating so that you can experience the taste and texture of the food/drink.
- Sit down. Make somewhat of a ceremony or ritual of eating. It can be a pleasant activity in and of itself rather than a side event to whatever else you are doing.
- Make the food look appetizing, as we eat with our eyes too. Think about a meal you had at a lovely restaurant and how it was served to you.
- Make sure there are no distractions. Put your phone away and turn off the television.
- Set yourself a goal of one or two mouthfuls instead of the whole meal to practise eating mindfully.

Feel free to give this a go with your next meal. If you'd like to practise this in a gradual way, however, you might like to start with a food that has a lot of sensory experiences you can pay attention to.

Remember, mindfulness is about the process, not the outcome. It is not about being a master or being "perfect" at it, but about the practice. If you are prone to focusing on outcomes and doing things perfectly, read on.

CHAPTER 19

THE PROBLEM WITH PERFECTIONISM

Trying our best to achieve high standards in what we do can be a positive attribute. High standards might help us to do well in life and they are rewarded by society, both economically and socially. However, when these standards become unrelenting, rigid and you are unable to cope with not meeting them, things become problematic. In their book, *Overcoming Perfectionism*, Roz Shafran and colleagues list the following three features of perfectionism[11]:

- Demanding standards and self-criticism
- Striving to meet these standards despite the consequences
- Basing self-evaluation on these standards

People with eating problems are prone to perfectionism. This is not surprising given that we have looked at the role of strict diet rules, or of striving for the so-called "perfect" body. You might have become caught in striving for this unrealistic "perfect" image via eating "cleaner", detoxing and exercising frequently, perpetuating the idea that this standard is possible.

As perfectionism tends to be part of our broader personality style, if you are perfectionistic about eating or your body, you are probably perfectionistic in other areas of your life, such as work or relationships. If this is you, you might strive to be the perfect

---

[11] Shafran, R., Egan, S. & Wade, T. (2010). *Overcoming perfectionism: A self-help guide using scientifically supported cognitive behavioral techniques.* Robinson Publishing: London, UK.

partner – for example, believing that your partner will not be attracted to you if you don't dress in the perfect way. Similarly, in the work environment, you may have demanding standards related to productivity or career progression, and if you do not meet 100% of your targets you think you have failed. Or you might excessively berate yourself if you make a mistake.

The problem is, pursuing these extremely high standards sets you up for disappointment and more extreme expectations when you have not met your standards. Extremely high standards are almost always impossible to achieve. The cost of having them is that you will likely never feel good enough. This, in turn, will lead to greater disappointment, feelings of failure, self-criticism and increased anxiety. Making mistakes is all part of being human, and it is often through making mistakes that we learn and enrich our lives.

> "Extremely high standards are almost always impossible to achieve. The cost of having them is that you will likely never feel good enough."

SIGNS OF PERFECTIONISM

The following are signs of perfectionism. Which ones can you relate to?

- Difficulty making decisions in time
- Constantly organising
- Procrastinating due to worry that it won't be good enough
- Being overinclusive with detail
- Excessive checking
- Avoiding situations where there is a possibility of failing
- Dwelling on mistakes
- Having to start a task from the beginning if a small error is made
- Seeking reassurance but not feeling reassured

Despite what you may believe, perfectionism does not actually help you to achieve more. When striving for something, an element of stress and pressure helps to focus us. However, too much stress and pressure tends to overwhelm us and leads to lower performance and to procrastination. Not to mention, the cost of having these standards will probably mean you are a high achiever who is miserable, stressed and thinking that you are never good enough. On balance, what is more important?

EXAMINE YOUR THINKING

If you find yourself in a cycle of perfectionistic thoughts and behaviours, ask yourself: would it be so bad if things were not 100% perfect? What are you really afraid of? Perhaps you worry that people will think you are deficient in some way, or that you will let others down. Maybe you worry that others will not like you if you are not perfect. Have a think about what is underlying this pattern of thinking for you. Just like food rules, what performance rules are you caught striving to live by? For example, "I must not make a mistake or I'll be judged"? "I must always aim for perfection or I'll be a failure"?

Go back to the chapters on thought challenging and think about what might be a healthier rule, or a healthier thought about yourself. Look over the unhelpful thinking styles, for example black-and-white thinking, personalisation or should-ing/must-ing, and ask yourself: "Am I engaging in an unhelpful thinking style again?"

Often people are afraid that if they let go of perfectionistic expectations, the alternative is they will aim for nothing and therefore achieve nothing. Try to be balanced in any alternative you come up with. Letting go of perfectionism does not mean

"Letting go of perfectionism does not mean you let go of all ambition! It just means you take a more reasonable approach with yourself."

you let go of all ambition! It just means you take a more reasonable approach with yourself.

TEST YOUR BEHAVIOUR

Could you aim to be "good enough" or average in some domains of your life? Think about how you might be able to test out your rules or predictions about being imperfect. If you think that by making a mistake, others will think you are inadequate, try it out. Notice your perfectionistic behaviours and try to slowly reduce them. If you find yourself looking in the mirror for many hours a day checking if your appearance is "just right", try to reduce the amount of time you spend doing this. If you avoid speaking up with your friends or colleagues because you worry that you won't get your point out perfectly enough, give it a go. You might think that others will judge you, but actually it's possible they would like to know your perspective. What's more, they might share it.

"Remember: you are more than what you achieve!"

Maybe you could even make a mistake on purpose! This probably seems a strange thing to do, but by experimenting with this you may just find that your worst fear does not come to pass. Instead, you might be pleasantly surprised. Others could feel more endeared or even warm to you more as they could see this as a sign you are human and relatable. Who knows? There is only one way to find out...

ENLARGE YOUR VIEW

Achievement might be something that is really important to you. Perhaps take some time to think about the other things that are important to you and contribute to your sense of self-worth. Consider other qualities you have, such as being a kind friend, a loyal partner, a supportive parent, being funny, being talented at art or being a good listener. Try not to pin all of how you see yourself on your achievements. By doing that, you are marginalising all of the other domains in your life that give you meaning. Remember: you are more than what you achieve!

Perfectionism is common among those who struggle with eating problems. We have already looked at how strict, unrealistic eating and body-related goals can fuel eating problems, and in this chapter we have discovered that unrealistic perfectionistic goals can also fuel eating problems. Although perfectionistic striving is usually intended to better yourself, it has the unintended effect of causing distress and leading to poor self-esteem. Read on as we touch on self-esteem and how this can be an obstacle to tackling your eating problems.

CHAPTER 20

FOSTERING SELF-ESTEEM

Eating problems are often related to a poor view of oneself, sometimes known as low self-esteem. As we have discussed, many people, for one reason or another, hold a belief that they are a failure or not good enough. Patterns of dieting, exercise and focusing on your body are often strategies people use to try to enhance their self-worth and feel acceptable. However, the inevitable breaking of diet rules and binge eating, or not reaching shape and weight ideals, only serves to make them feel worse.

If this sounds like you, to truly let go of your eating problems you will need to work on how you view yourself as a whole person. Keep reading below to see what we mean.

SELF-CRITICISM

Within us, we all have an inner critical voice. Sometimes it's helpful and we need it. Sometimes, however, this critic can become out of control and begin to criticise too often and too harshly. This experience of an overly harsh inner critic is commonly related to eating problems. The inner voice might say black-and-white things like "You're not good enough," "You're greedy," "Your friends don't really like you" or "You're hopeless – you'll never get over this problem." Do you recognise these thoughts, or this tone of speaking? If so, it's important to notice this inner critic and the impact it is having on you.

These types of statements tend to have a detrimental impact on your happiness, wellbeing and the energy and motivation you need for your goals. They will wear you down and continue to erode your sense of self-worth. Living with a voice like this is exhausting. If you recognise that you take this approach with yourself, then we hope that you will take a moment now to have some compassion with yourself for living with such a harsh inner critic. We doubt that you would want to speak to a friend this way, so why talk to yourself this way?

"Have some compassion with yourself for living with such a harsh inner critic. We doubt that you would want to speak to a friend this way, so why talk to yourself this way?"

If you struggle with high levels of self-criticism, here are some ideas for the way forward.

NOTICE IT

When you reflect on your journal, keep an additional look out for the harsh critic. Go back through your writing and circle any statements you notice that, in retrospect, could be the voice of the critic. If you want some more help identifying it (as sometimes it can feel more "who you are" rather than just a part of your mindset), then you might want to ask a friend to help. We also recommend you keep an eye out for "shoulds" and notice what you are "should-ing" yourself into. The critic loves to latch on to an unreasonable "should"! It also loves to label – saying that you as a person are *globally bad* because of something that went wrong in a particular situation. See if you can notice those labels. For more information about what to look out for in noticing your inner critic, check out the book *Self-Esteem* by McKay and Fanning (2016).

WEIGH UP THE COSTS AND BENEFITS OF THIS APPROACH

Like all other issues we've discussed, we think this experience of criticising yourself happens for a reason. Nobody *wants* to berate themselves and make themselves feel awful, unless they believe it does something good. Ask yourself:

- What am I trying to achieve by berating myself in this way? Do I believe that it will help me achieve more?
- Do I believe that if I criticise myself first, I'll be prepared for other's criticisms?
- Is self-criticism really working to help me with my goals?
- What are the costs of listening to this harsh inner critic?

Even if your self-criticism motivates you to achieve, we have often seen that this still leads to people feeling miserable and scared. You might like to spend some time writing down the pros and cons of continuing to listen to this critic, to see what reasons you might be holding on to it.

BE BALANCED

Once you've noticed the critic, you have created a moment to choose how to respond. Noticing gives you options. You can choose to challenge the critic and talk back with a more reasonable statement. Or you can ask yourself what you would say to a friend in the same situation. It is likely to be more reasonable!

Often the statements are global criticisms of you (or others) as a person. If so, try to take a balanced approach with yourself. We all have strengths and weaknesses. Focusing exclusively on either one is likely to lead to problems. Instead, acknowledge that you are more than your behaviour in one situation, and you are more than one of your characteristics.

LET GO

Often, a harsh inner critic repeats the same statements over and over and over again – never giving you new information, just repeating how bad you are. Even if you know it's not true, this can really wear you down. If this is the case, check out our section on over-thinking for some ideas about how to get some distance from the critic. Tell yourself, "There's that critic again," and let it go.

SHAME

Shame is the feeling linked to a belief about ourselves as globally bad and is often linked to a sense of being unacceptable to others. As humans we all *need* to be socially connected with others, so anything that brings up feelings of shame seems threatening due to the risk of being disconnected.

Because shame feels so deeply threatening, we naturally want to push it away. Eating problems are a way to manage this complex and difficult emotion. Unfortunately, like other feelings and thoughts, avoiding shame, rather than working through it, will create more problems for you.

Finding healthy ways to respond to shame is a challenge for all of us. Some approaches that might help include:

COMPASSION

An antidote to shame is compassion. Compassion is defined by expert Dr Kristin Neff[12] as having three key components:

1) Being kind to yourself rather than judging yourself

2) A sense of "common humanity" – recognising we are all in this together, as opposed to thinking, "This is only me" or "I'm on my own".

---

12 Neff, K. (2020). *Definition of Self-Compassion*. Available at: self-compassion.org/the-three-elements-of-self-compassion-2 [Accessed 30 July 2020].

3) Being mindful of your negative experiences, *observing* them with openness, rather than over-identifying with and becoming swept up in them.

Remind yourself that it is *understandable* that you have come to be in the place you are. You did not choose the life you have

"Next time you feel shame and an urge to turn to your eating problem, see if you can catch yourself and instead show yourself some compassion."

been thrown into, but you can choose now how to respond to the place you are in. Next time you feel an urge to use a problem eating behaviour to cope with feelings of shame, see if you can catch yourself and instead show yourself some compassion.

ACCEPT YOURSELF AS "GOOD ENOUGH"

Shame can arise when you negatively judge your *entire* worth based on imperfections that are *wholly normal and universally experienced* – such as mistakes, flaws and misfortunes. If you think you're only worthy (and others will see you as worthy) for meeting certain requirements, then you're prone to feel shame more often. Proactively work on being accepting of yourself as *good enough as you are*, with strengths and weaknesses like all human beings.

AUTHENTICITY

Shame is often a social emotion and it is common to want to *bury* your shame in an effort not to be exposed. The thing is, the more we hide ourselves from one another, the more "strange" and "wrong" we each feel, as we don't realise others are struggling with the same things as us! Being authentic with (chosen) others, sharing your vulnerabilities and fears, can take the heat out of shame-provoking experiences, and can help you truly connect with others. If you begin to open up with others, you will find that some of the things you feel ashamed about

> "Shame can arise when you negatively judge your entire worth based on imperfections that are wholly normal and universally experienced – such as mistakes, flaws and misfortunes."

are actually more common than you think! Realising this tends to defuse shame. If you are interested in this issue, we highly recommend *The Gifts of Imperfection* by Brené Brown (2010).

We have only briefly touched on self-esteem and shame in this chapter, because it is beyond the scope of this book. However, if these points are relevant for you and your eating problems, we strongly advise you to seek out some of the recommended literature.

We hope this chapter has given you an opportunity to reflect on how you see and relate to yourself, and to notice if you are highly critical or shaming of yourself. How we relate to ourselves inevitably impacts on how we relate to others. In the next chapter we will look more at this.

CHAPTER 21

RELATIONSHIPS

We are social creatures and relationships are important. Difficulties in relationships can make you more vulnerable to eating problems, and, at the same time, eating problems can have a big impact on your relationships. Exploring your relational style and how this might be connected with your eating problems might be key to lasting change.

We now discuss the issues in relationships that might arise and could be having an impact on your eating problem.

PRIORITISING OTHERS AND NEGLECTING YOURSELF

As you may have gathered, improving your relationship with food has to be a priority for you. This can be a problem when you tend to prioritise others before yourself. While it's okay to care for others, a pattern of always focusing on others' needs means you neglect yourself (and perhaps then neglect your body's needs and your nutritional needs). This could leave you feeling frustrated and resentful. If this is you, ask yourself: is this how you want to continue? Or could you treat yourself with the same understanding and care that you are treating others? Remember that your value is equal to theirs.

"While it's okay to care for others, a pattern of always focusing on others' needs means you neglect yourself."

COMMUNICATION DIFFICULTIES

Many people with eating problems are afraid to open up due to a variety of fears. You may have developed a belief that being emotional or vulnerable will lead to people not liking you. Or a belief that if you are anything less than perfect, you will be rejected. If so, it's likely that you struggle to share your honest problems with others, which may leave you feeling quite alone or stressed.

In this situation you may find yourself trying to communicate how you feel via your eating behaviour. Perhaps if you skip a meal there is an underlying hope that someone will notice and ask how you are? Or if you obsessively exercise, that somebody will praise you and you will feel the connection and acceptance that you are craving?

The difficulty is that communicating in this indirect way won't get your true needs met. It is also likely that your need won't be understood; you might get sympathy rather than connection, or might only be acknowledged temporarily, which will leave you feeling even worse. In addition, this communication style might hamper your chances to learn other, more effective ways of relating to others.

We all find ourselves communicating in indirect ways at times. If this is a pattern for you, consider if you could be willing to risk talking openly with others, communicating in a more direct, assertive way in order to get your true needs met.

RELYING ON OTHERS FOR A SENSE OF WORTH

You may have a belief that you are only acceptable if others deem you acceptable. However, attaching a prerequisite of others' acceptance to your sense of worth makes your self-esteem vulnerable. Thinking, "If others accept me, I'm worthy" puts you in a difficult place as it leaves you at the mercy of your *perception* of others' judgements, which you can never fully know.

It also leaves you focused on meeting others' priorities in life, rather than your own. We think that to feel most satisfied in your own life, it is important to focus on living according to _your_ values and goals.

If this is you, remind yourself right now that you are a worthy and acceptable individual. Foster that belief. By doing so, you will be less _preoccupied_ with pleasing others and being accepted by them, and have more mental and emotional space to focus on enjoying the relationship as it is.

Relationships are central to our existence as humans. You are not alone in this world and meaningful equal relationships are important and possible. Feeling good in yourself, and good in your relationships helps to set the foundation for a positive relationship with your body and food. This will help in overcoming eating problems in a lasting way.

> "Thinking, 'If others accept me, I'm worthy' puts you in a difficult place as it leaves you at the mercy of your perception of others' judgements, which you can never fully know."

CHAPTER 22

KEEP GOING

You have made it! Hopefully, by now you feel equipped and ready to carve out a new path free of eating problems. Of course, if you have struggled for a long time, it will not be that simple and your motivation, confidence and ability to make and practise the necessary changes may wax and wane. This is normal and, as always, try to bring an attitude of self-compassion to this new path. In any case, we hope that you now feel ready to carry on this new and exciting journey.

"Change is rarely linear."

REFLECT ON YOUR PROGRESS

You may have already made significant changes to your eating. Or you may have read through this book at speed, know the path forward, but are still part-way through the journey away from your eating problems.

Change is rarely linear. Often people describe taking two steps forward, then one back. The process of moving forward tends to look like this:

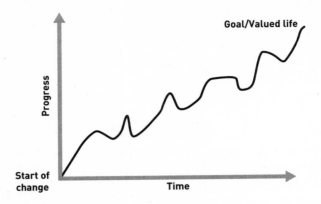

Whatever point you are at, it is important to reflect back on the journey and look at what you have achieved, what has helped so far, and what you would still like to change. It can help to draw this graph and ask yourself:

- Where am I on the journey at this point?
- What changes have I made?
- What has helped me make these changes?
- What changes would I still like to make?
- What are obstacles that are getting in the way of making change?
- What techniques or skills could I use to tackle these obstacles?

WHAT HAS HELPED

Go through the parts of the book that really resonated with you. We expect that there will be some things that felt more relevant than others. That's okay. Just go back to what you connected with and think about how you can practise the skills and make these changes.

Summarise the points that you found most helpful below and find a place you can keep these points nearby. As we have said, if you truly want to change your behaviour, then practice is the key. Practise what has helped already – whether that be your alternative thoughts, regular eating, testing your beliefs, gratitude towards your body, mindfulness or any of the techniques mentioned in this book.

EXERCISE: LOOKING BACK

What are the things I need to remind myself in order to keep improving my relationship with food? What are the practical steps I can take?

BE PREPARED

Like any journey, keep a map of where you are heading. Remember the values we discussed early on and use these to orientate you forward.

In order to stay on track, we encourage you to think about the early indicators that you might be going off track. These might include cutting out certain food groups, or perhaps not taking time out to practise self-care. It could be that you have abandoned regular eating or maybe you are weighing yourself more often.

"Blips are normal and are not a sign of a complete relapse."

Also hold in mind the situations that increase your urge to return to problem eating behaviours. This will be individual to you, but common situations that increase the pull to eating problems include

> **"Try to catch the problem as soon as you can. Early intervention is key to making change easier."**

tiredness, increased social media usage, or work stress. Whatever the case, try to be switched on to individual signs and indicators relevant to you to help prevent blips.

If you notice these happening, try to catch the problem as soon as you can. Early intervention is key to making change easier.

DEALING WITH BLIPS

It is common when we are changing our behaviour to fall back into old patterns sometimes. The same goes with eating problems. If you notice that you have started to revert back to your old ways, try to see this as a *blip* rather than a sign that you are back at the beginning again. Blips are normal and are not a sign of a complete relapse. When you notice one, congratulate yourself first for noticing it. It is great progress to even be aware of the blip! Then come back to the points above to help orient you back on the journey. Try to do this sooner rather than later.

Ups and downs are a normal part of life. Sometimes we notice people on the path to an improved relationship with food and their bodies expect smooth sailing. In our experience, however, this is rarely the case. Sometimes people respond to a blip with self-criticism or even the "Sod it" or "I give up" effect. Both of these responses will likely make recovery so much harder in the long run.

> **"Remember: you are learning a whole new way of coping with food, your body, and probably your emotions. Be kind to yourself."**

If your inclination is to be overly hard on yourself, we encourage you to remember how far you have come and try to bring some self-compassion to the situation. What would you tell a friend if they were trying a new way of eating or engaging with their emotions, and they momentarily fell into old habits? We are sure that you would not berate them or criticise their lack of effort or their actions. So, try not to catastrophise, criticise yourself, or feel hopeless. See a blip as a chance to learn about what situations continue to be difficult and see each moment of a day as an opportunity to return again to the new road you're on. Try to use the techniques covered in this book to reorientate and get back on the path away from your eating problems. Remember: you are learning a whole new way of coping with food, your body, and probably your emotions. Be kind to yourself.

SEEK FACE-TO-FACE SUPPORT

As already mentioned, this book is not meant to substitute professional face-to-face therapy if this is what is required. You may find that you still are struggling with your eating despite giving the strategies in this book a good go. Or you might notice that underlying your eating problems are other issues related to your mood and anxiety, relationships or self-esteem, for which you need more intense support. If this is you, we recommend you find the professional body in your area that represents Psychologists or Cognitive Behavioural Therapists. Look for a registered clinician that has specialist experience in treating eating problems.

A STORY OF HOPE

For years, "Suzy" struggled with eating problems and preoccupying shape and weight concerns. She tells such an amazing story of the process and outcome of her journey to encourage you all. Unlike the other characters in this book, Suzy is a real person who chooses to remain anonymous but who has kindly contributed her story. It is a powerful reminder that change is possible and totally worth it.

I can still remember the first "diet" I went on. I was 16 years old and a friend and I started an apple, cheese, chicken and salad diet. For two days you'd eat nothing but apples, then for two days nothing but cheese, followed by two days eating nothing but chicken and finally two days nothing but salad. On the seventh day, you'd have lost a ton of weight. We failed on day 4.

The next time I went on a diet I was following in the footsteps of what sounded like a credible, science-based celebrity diet. I made it through a few weeks of serious undereating then spectacularly vomited Diet Coke and vodka all over my best friend's bed after an evening of attempted drinking. Apparently in my drunken state I confessed to her, crying, that I just wanted to lose weight. She took me straight to Burger King.

I wanted to weigh the same amount I'd read a fashionable celebrity I'd begun to idolise did. I kept a folder hidden in my computer files with photos of her or other tiny women that I would use as motivation for myself to one day look like them.

I was only eighteen years old and already absolutely convinced about the importance in life of being thin.

It took me over a decade to admit that I had a problem, that I needed help, and that I needed to change. What was my problem? Preoccupation with my body image and attempting to control the size of my body by controlling my food intake.

There's a lot of reasons it took me so long to confront the issues. The first is because, as far as I could tell, everybody was preoccupied with body image and attempting to control their weight through diet. Media confirmed this, overhearing snippets of conversations between strangers confirmed this, and – most sadly of all – many of my closest friends' attitudes confirmed this, which to me meant that if I did have any type of a problem, it was certainly one that was normal, so couldn't be that bad.

Now that I've recovered, I can tell you one thing for sure: not everybody suffers from these problems and the fact that so many people do doesn't mean it should be considered normal. It means that as a problem I think it urgently needs fixing – both for individuals and on a larger scale, as a shift in cultural paradigm.

I won't go into all of the details of what the years of problem eating involved for me – everybody's story is different – but what I'd like to share with you is what led me to finally make some changes, and to let you know that it is possible to confront these problems and to enjoy your life liberated from the chains of problem eating.

I finally sought help when I was 30 years old – twelve years after the Diet Coke vomit bed incident.

In my more recent years, any problems I had with eating had been successfully masked as a resolve to live a "healthy" lifestyle. I'd been able to control my weight through a combination of excessive exercise and "clean eating", including regularly completing a super low-calorie diet I'd found online that promised weight loss results in just seven days.

I felt I was doing pretty well as I hadn't abused laxatives in about nine years, and even though I was still checking the size of my stomach 10–20 times a day since I'd taken up a rigorous exercise regime and a protein smoothie diet, these checks only offered me reassurance that I could still see the outline of my abs. I also consumed a daily "fat burning" supplement that kept my hunger pangs in check. But so did nearly everyone I knew in the gym world at the time.

Then I went through a painful divorce. I moved to London. And the scale of my problem slowly got worse. I started to put on weight again. Which *terrified me. So I'd vow to lose it. Binge. Restrict. Binge. Restrict. Binge. Restrict. I felt out of control and absolutely fed up.*

There wasn't any one single defining moment when I realised something needed to change. It wasn't like a lightbulb turning on. Instead, the sheer exhaustion finally overcame me. I felt tired to my bones. Tired of trying to stick to a diet. Of failing over and over again. Tired of taking "before" photos of my body and staring at them in shame. Tired of placing such a high importance on my weight. I thought to myself: do I really want to be obsessing over this for all my years to come?

I didn't. I wanted to be like the people I knew who cared about other stuff. Who invested their energy into things that brought them joy, not misery. I wanted eating to just be something I could do… normally. But it had been so long I genuinely didn't know what normal eating even was.

And so I started the process of examining my thoughts. Examining my behaviours around food. I made notes in my journal. I analysed myself without judgement. I spoke with a therapist. I confided in close friends and family. I started to pursue goals that were important to me. And I committed to eating regularly.

Only a year or so after starting this journey of change, I was sitting in a café eating a large piece of carrot cake and I was smiling as I ate. I was finding it delicious, which made me happy, but so much more than that. It dawned on me that the old thought patterns hadn't occurred. I didn't analyse the calories, didn't panic about the sugar content, didn't think about skipping dinner or criticise myself for my lack of self-control. It was a moment I could have only dreamed of before.

It's worth it to change, and when you experience moments like those for yourself, it feels so good to be free.

USEFUL RESOURCES

In the UK, if you wish to access individual therapy, the first port of call is to request an NHS referral via your GP to either general mental health services or specialist eating disorder services. You can also self-refer to your local Improving Access to Psychological Therapy (IAPT) service. IAPT provides more general talking therapies. If you are under the age of 18, they may also refer you to your local specialist Child and Adolescent Eating Disorder Service (CAMHS).

For private therapists, there is list on the BEAT website: www.beateatingdisorders.org.uk/ or on the BPS www.bps.org.uk/public/find-psychologist or BACP website www.bacp.co.uk/. We recommend that you find a therapist that is registered with a professional body as this ensures professional accountability and integrity. For private registered dietitians specialising in eating disorders and disordered eating, you can find them listed on the BEAT website or the Freelance Dietitians website freelancedietitians.org/dietitians-in-private-practice.

RECOMMENDED READING

In addition to this, and if you are based elsewhere, there are many books and resources that have inspired us in our practice. See below for our recommended reading, which we hope could be an extra resource to you.

EATING-RELATED

Bacon, L. (2010). *Health at Every Size: The surprising truth about your weight*. BenBella Books: Dallas, TX, US.

Cash, T. (2008). *Body Image Workbook: An Eight-step Program for Learning to Like Your Looks*. New Harbinger: Oakland, CA, US.

Fairburn, C.G. (2013). *Overcoming Binge Eating* (2nd ed). Guilford Press: New York, NY, US.

Gilbert, P. (2010). *The Compassionate mind*. Constable: London, UK.

Goldacre, B. (2009). Bad Science. Fourth Estate: London, UK.

Goss, K. (2011). *Beating Overeating: Using compassion focused therapy*. Robinson Publishing: London, UK.

Schmidt, U., Treasure, J., & Alexander, J. (2015). *Getting Better Bit(e) by Bit(e): A Survival Kit for Sufferers of Bulimia Nervosa and Binge Eating Disorders*. Routledge: London, UK.

Thomas, L. (2019). *Just Eat It*. Bluebird Publishing: London, UK.

Tribole, E. & Resch, E. (2012). *Intuitive Eating: A revolutionary program that works*. St. Martin's Griffin: New York, NY, US.

Waller, G., Mountford, V., Lawson, R., Gray, E., Cordery, H & Hinrichsen, H. (2010). *Beating your eating disorder: A cognitive behavioural self-help guide for adult sufferers and their carers*. Cambridge University Press: Cambridge, UK.

RELATED ISSUES

Brown, B. (2010). *The Gifts of Imperfection: Let Go of Who You Think You're Supposed to Be and Embrace Who You Are*. Hazelden Publishing: Center City, MN, US.

Burns, D. (1998). *Feeling Good: The New Mood Therapy*. Avon Books: New York, NY, US.

Greenberger, D. & Padesky, C. (2015). *Mind Over Mood: Change How You Feel by Changing the Way You Think 2nd Edition*. Guilford Press: New York, NY, US.

McKay, M. & Fanning, P. (2016). *Self-Esteem, 4th Edition: A Proven Program of Cognitive Techniques for Assessing, Improving, and Maintaining your Self-Esteem*. New Harbinger: Oakland, CA, US.

Shafran, ER., Egan, S., & Wade, T. (2018). *Overcoming Perfectionism 2nd Edition: A self-help guide using scientifically supported cognitive behavioural techniques*. Robinson Publishing: London, UK.

Young, J. & Klosko, J. (2019). *Reinventing your Life: The breakthrough program to end negative behaviour and feel great again: the breakthrough programme to end negative behaviour and feel great again*. Scribe Publications: London, UK.

Williams, M. & Penny, D. (2011). *Mindfulness: A practical guide to Finding Peace in a Frantic World*. Piatkus: London, UK.

CARERS RESOURCES

Treasure, J., Smith, G., & Crane, A. (2016). *Skills-based caring for a loved one with an eating disorder: The new Maudsley method* (2nd ed). Routledge: London, UK.

CLINICIAN RESOURCES

Fairburn, C. (2008). *Cognitive Behavior Therapy and Eating Disorders*. Guilford Press: New York, NY, US.

Waller, G., Cordery, H., Corstorphine, E., Hinrichsen, H., Lawson, R., Mountford, V., & Russell, K. (2007). *Cognitive behavioral therapy for eating disorders: A comprehensive treatment guide*. Cambridge University Press: Cambridge, UK.

USEFUL WEBSITES

Centre for Clinical Interventions: www.cci.health.wa.gov.au. This website has a number of useful self-help resources. The ones we find particularly relevant in relation to eating problems include workbooks on "Disordered Eating" and "Appearance Concerns". There are also a range of further workbooks to help with related problems such as perfectionism, anxiety or tolerating distress.

BEAT: www.beateatingdisorders.org.uk. This website is for a UK-based charity offering guidance and support related to eating disorders.

National Eating Disorders Association: www. nationaleatingdisorders.org. This website is a US-based eating disorders charity.

Eating Disorder Hope: www.eatingdisorderhope.com/ treatment-for-eating-disorders/international/australia/australias-eating-disorder-organizations-charities. This is an Australian-based eating disorders charity.

USEFUL APPS

There are an abundance of useful apps available to help with eating, anxiety, emotions, relaxation, mindfulness and general wellbeing. Here are three of our favourites, but we recommend you spend some time finding those that work for you.

Recovery Record – an eating disorder recovery app

Headspace – a mindfulness and relaxation app

Calm – an anxiety, mindfulness and relaxation app

ABOUT TRIGGER PUBLISHING

Trigger is a leading independent altruistic global publisher devoted to opening up conversations about mental health and wellbeing. We share uplifting and inspirational mental health stories, publish advice-driven books by highly qualified clinicians for those in recovery and produce wellbeing books that will help you to live your life with greater meaning and clarity.

Founder Adam Shaw, mental health advocate and philanthropist, established the company with leading psychologist Lauren Callaghan, whilst in recovery from serious mental health issues. Their aim was to publish books which provided advice and support to anyone suffering with mental illness by sharing uplifting and inspiring stories from real-life survivors, combined with expert advice on practical recovery techniques.

Since then, Trigger has expanded to produce books on a wide range of topics surrounding mental health and wellness, as well as launching *Upside Down*, its children's list, which encourages open conversation around mental health from a young age.

We want to help you to not just survive but thrive ... one book at a time.

Find out more about Trigger Publishing by visiting our website:triggerpublishing.com or join us on:

Twitter @TriggerPub

Facebook @TriggerPub

Instagram @TriggerPub

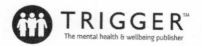

ABOUT SHAW MIND

A proportion of profits from the sale of all Trigger books go to their sister charity, Shaw Mind, also founded by Adam Shaw and Lauren Callaghan. The charity aims to ensure that everyone has access to mental health resources whenever they need them.

You can find out more about the work that Shaw Mind do by visiting their website: shawmindfoundation.org or joining them on
Twitter: @Shaw_Mind
Instagram: @Shaw_Mind
LinkedIn: @shaw-mind
Facebook: @shawmindUK

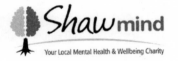

Your Local Mental Health & Wellbeing Charity